Men's Health

Life Improvement Guides™

Powerfully Fit

Dozens of Ways
to Boost Strength, Increase
Endurance and Chisel
Your Body

by Brian Chichester, Jack Croft
and the Editors of Men'sHealth Books

Rodale Press, Inc.
Emmaus, Pennsylvania

Copyright © 1996 by Rodale Press, Inc.

Cover photograph copyright © 1996 by Mitch Mandel/RSI
Illustrations copyright © 1996 by Mark Matcho

Printed in the United States of America on acid-free (∞), recycled paper ♻

Other titles in the *Men's Health Life Improvement Guides* series:

Fight Fat	*Stress Blasters*
Food Smart	*Symptom Solver*
Sex Secrets	

Library of Congress Cataloging-in-Publication Data

Chichester, Brian.
    Powerfully fit : dozens of ways to boost strength,
increase endurance and chisel your body / by Brian Chichester,
Jack Croft and the editors of Men's Health Books.
      p.   cm. — (Men's health life improvement guides)
    Includes index.
    ISBN 0–87596–279–3 paperback
    1. Physical fitness for men.   2. Exercise for men.
3. Muscle strength. I. Croft, Jack. II. Men's Health Books.
III. Title. IV. Series.
GV482.5.C55 1996
613.7′0449—dc20   95–25484

Distributed in the book trade by St. Martin's Press

  4 6 8 10 9 7 5   paperback

OUR PURPOSE

*"We inspire and enable people to improve
their lives and the world around them."*

Powerfully Fit Editorial Staff
Senior Managing Editor: **Neil Wertheimer**
Senior Editor: **Jack Croft**
Writers: **Brian Chichester, Jack Croft, Jeff Bredenberg, Stephen C. George**
Book and Cover Designer: **John Herr**
Cover Photographer: **Mitch Mandel**
Photo Editor: **Susan Pollack**
Illustrators: **Mark Matcho, John Herr**
Studio Manager: **Joe Golden**
Technical Artists: **William L. Allen, David Q. Pryor**
Assistant Research Manager: **Carlotta Cuerdon**
Researchers and Fact-Checkers: **Jan Eickmeier, Theresa Fogarty, Deborah Pedron, Sally A. Reith, John Waldron**
Copy Editor: **Amy K. Fisher**
Production Manager: **Helen Clogston**
Manufacturing Coordinator: **Jodi Schaffer**
Office Staff: **Roberta Mulliner, Julie Kehs, Bernadette Sauerwine, Mary Lou Stephen**

Rodale Health and Fitness Books
Vice-President and Editorial Director: **Debora T. Yost**
Art Director: **Jane Colby Knutila**
Research Manager: **Ann Gossy Yermish**
Copy Manager: **Lisa D. Andruscavage**

Photo Credits
Cover and all photographs by **Mitch Mandel/RSI** except those listed below.
Page 142: **Tim Hancock/Sports File**
Page 144: **Donna Chiarelli**
Page 146: **John Huet**
Page 148: **Carey Frame**
Page 150: **Allsport/Clive Brunskill**
Page 152: **Robert Oliver**
Page 154: **Pulak Viscardi**
Back flap: **Brown Brothers**

Contents

Part Five

The Perfect Exercise

Part Six

Real-Life Scenarios

Power Routines

Quest for the Best

You Can Do It!

Introduction

Navigating the Road to Power

Becoming powerfully fit is hard work. So we've done our best to make sure that reading *Powerfully Fit* isn't.

Our book's premise is simple: Whatever you do in life, weight training can help you do it better. This guide is jam-packed with all the information you need to launch a successful weight-training program—or take your current workout to the next level.

What separates *Powerfully Fit* from other fitness books is that this one helps you design a program to accomplish your own unique goals. Whether you want to build a rippling body that turns heads, increase your stamina for longer bike rides or just be able to spend Saturday working in the garden without having to spend Sunday nursing sore muscles, this book is your personal guide.

In Part One: The Road to Power, you'll find the very latest scientific information on the amazing benefits offered by resistance training. You'll discover helpful tips on everything from the best foods for fueling your muscle machine to how to avoid injuries and stay motivated.

Part Two: Power Where You Need It shows you how to do dozens of exercises the right way. This is the map you'll turn to again and again during your journey on the road to power. It's conveniently broken down by the specific areas of your body you want to work. Just about every exercise you need to know is carefully illustrated and explained. They are all grouped together so you always know where to turn for a quick and easy refresher course. And after you've mastered the basics, you might want to move up to *The Next Level*—a series of more challenging exercises intended for serious weight lifters.

In the next two sections you'll learn which exercises you need to do for specific activities. Part Three: Power at Play teaches exercises that will give you the edge in sports ranging from running to bowling to skiing. Part Four: Real-Life Power is your guide to building strength for everything from great sex to lifting heavy objects.

In Part Five: The Perfect Exercise, we'll show you the correct way to do basic exercises such as push-ups, crunches and jumping rope.

Finally, we bring it all together in Part Six: Real-Life Scenarios. If you want to lift weights to improve your general health, we'll tell you how. If you want to sculpt your body into a living portrait of power, you'll find the program here. If your goal is to be able to run or bike further without fatigue, it's all here. And if you want to become more flexible, we have a program for that, too. For inspiration, world-class athletes like Olympic gold-medal skier Tommy Moe and tennis great Michael Chang share their training secrets. And you'll also find profiles and tips from regular guys—just like you—who have become powerfully fit.

One final thought: This book may look great on your bookshelf, but it doesn't really belong there. It belongs in your basement, garage or local gym—wherever you go to work out. Sure, it's informative, entertaining and a helluva good read—that's the point of all the *Men's Health* Life Improvement Guides. But it's meant to be used, to guide you as you transform your body into a powerfully fit machine.

Have a great trip.

Neil Wertheimer
Senior Managing Editor, *Men's Health* Books

Part One

The Road to Power

What Is Physical Power?

To Work and Play Better, Join the Resistance

You flip through computer magazines and salivate over the latest mega-chips, the ones that would really kick byte in your home office.

Your stockbroker wheels around in a Corvette because he never knows when he'll need to roar from 0 to 60 mph in 5.2 seconds.

And rather than using a simple screwdriver, you rev up a thunderous, two-handled, half-inch drill to drive those four screws into the wall at 850 rpm.

Men adore power. Powerful machines work better, play better and look better. After all, which would you rather own: that sleek Corvette or a Volkswagen Beetle? The same principle applies to the most sophisticated machine you own—your body.

When you're powerfully fit, you can climb the jungle gym *with* your kids, rather than watching from the park bench. You can smash tennis balls far out of your opponent's reach. You can haul garden mulch until the sunlight—not your energy or your back—gives out. And you can have a T-shirt–optional kind of body on the beach.

Just a few years ago, if you decided to get yourself into shape, chances are you would just lace up the jogging shoes gathering dust in the back of your closet and head out the door. You may still want to hit the streets. But doctors and scientists now say aerobic exercise is not enough. To be all-around fit, you need to strengthen and maintain muscle, too, and that's done by resistance training—more commonly known as weight lifting.

"Anything that you lift, push or pull during daily activity will be made easier if you're in a strengthened state," says Wade A. Lillegard, M.D., director of the primary care sports medicine fellowship at the Uniformed Services University of the Health Sciences in Bethesda, Maryland. "Whether you're hauling groceries or climbing stairs, it just becomes less of a load on your system, particularly the heart."

Powerful Words

Men often equate power with brute strength. In basketball there are power forwards, players like Karl Malone who rip down rebounds and punish anyone who dares to drive the lane. The same standards apply in public life, where the late Richard J. Daley was often referred to as the most powerful mayor in the nation for the iron-fisted way he ran the Chicago political machine.

In scientific terms strength is certainly an integral part of power. But it's only half the equation. Muscular strength, as defined by scientists, is the amount of force a muscle group can exert. It's really a simple concept. Let's say the most you can bench-press one time is 100 pounds. Scientists call that a maximum voluntary contraction. Most of us call it plain old strength.

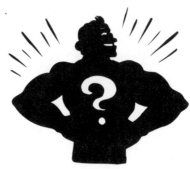

The concept of power, in scientific terms, goes a step further: It combines strength and speed. Power is the ability to move an object a certain distance in a certain amount of time. It's where your strength crosses over into practical life. Maybe you and your neighbor are able to wheelbarrow the same load of bricks 100 feet without stopping. But if you do it in half the time your neighbor took, then you're twice as powerful.

Muscle Growth: The Big Picture

Imagine driving your old Volkswagen Bug so long and hard that it evolves into a rip-roaring Porsche. Only one machine really works like that: the human body. When your muscles are consistently challenged by heavier resistance than they're used to, the first thing they do is get more efficient.

"There is a dramatic and almost immediate awakening of your brain talking to your muscles to say, 'I can lift something heavier than I have in the past,' and scientists call that neuromuscular control," says Wayne W. Campbell, Ph.D., an applied physiologist at Noll Physiological Research Center at Pennsylvania State University in University Park.

Most of your muscles are a combination of two basic types of fibers. Slow-twitch fibers are for endurance, the engine behind aerobic efforts such as long-distance running. Fast-twitch fibers provide the explosive force you need for sprints or bench presses. While most of us have about a 50-50 blend of slow- and fast-twitch muscle fibers, some folks are more genetically gifted one way or the other.

But the bottom line for most of us is that it's not what kind of muscle fiber you're born with that really counts. It's what you do with it that matters.

You have at your command more than 215 pairs of skeletal muscles, those that are lashed to your bones to make them move. At certain times in your life, you decide that you want more power in a specific movement—say, throwing a football. So you follow a strength-

Ride 'Em Longer, Cowboy

Tired of getting dirt in your teeth while trying to cling to large, crazed animals? Well, if you do it with muscles, you can do it better with *conditioned* muscles, and that applies to rodeo riding as surely as it does to football.

Researchers at the University of Wyoming in Laramie concluded that roughstock (bull, bareback and saddle bronc) riders would have more staying power and fewer injuries if they used resistance training to develop their legs, abdominals, lower back, shoulders, biceps and grip strength.

Exercise scientists measured the strength of collegiate roughstock riders, steer wrestlers, ropers and barrel racers. "We found that they were as strong as endurance athletes, but not as strong as power athletes," says researcher John G. Wilkinson, Ph.D. "Rodeo athletes are probably more like power athletes. They would need a whole-body conditioning program, because riding a relatively wild animal involves not only leg strength but upper-body strength as well."

ening routine, targeting the muscles that make that movement.

A routine that makes you a strong-armed quarterback, however, will do little for your bicycling career. To do effective resistance training, you must identify the muscle groups that are crucial for your chosen activity and then perform exercises that strengthen them. This is called the specificity principle.

To chart progress in a training program, each workout is broken down into repetitions (the number of times a weight is lifted), sets (groups of repetitions) and resistance (the amount of weight used).

The Heart's Role

Boosting Cardiovascular Power

Weight lifters like to work all the major muscles. But many of them miss one muscle that's among the most important in the body: the heart.

The two engines of your cardiovascular system are your heart and lungs. Their condition is an important benchmark of your overall health. Among the top benefits of a strong heart and lungs is stamina. "Cardiovascular training will give you the feel-good type of energy that can keep you going all day, even in the weight room," says Deborah Ellison, a physical therapist and fitness consultant in San Diego.

"It's especially important for men because men are at risk for heart problems, and weight training alone won't clean out your arteries," Ellison says.

Other Health Benefits

Building your cardiovascular system is a lot like building biceps. But instead of stressing muscle fiber with weight-lifting exercises, you're stressing your heart's ability to pump blood and your lungs' ability to provide oxygen with exercises that get you huffing and puffing. Most experts agree that in order to get the best cardiovascular (or "aerobic") workout, you should exercise hard enough to raise your pulse rate to 70 to 85 percent of your maximum, and then sustain that level for 20 minutes or more. A smart aerobic exercise routine would be at

least three times a week. Beginners aim for the 70 percent mark, fitter individuals the 85 percent mark.

Besides being able to climb a flight of stairs without asking for oxygen, having a healthy heart and lungs makes you powerful in other ways. The more aerobically fit you are, the less likely you are to have a heart attack or cardiovascular disease. Plus you'll rev your metabolism and torch fat in the process, which is always a healthy thing to do.

Lots of exercises can give you a cardiovascular edge: running, cycling, rowing, racquetball, basketball, hiking—anything that keeps your heart and lungs humming. You can even exercise your heart and lungs by working out your arms and chest, though the benefits of this are muted. Studies show that traditional aerobic exercises improve your lungs and heart power by about 18 percent, compared to 6 percent in a good fast-paced, high-rep weight-lifting regimen.

Weight Lifting and the Heart

Scientists are discovering that the payoff of resistance training can be similar to the payoff of cardiovascular exercise. Like aerobic exercise, weight lifting burns fat, lowers blood pressure and controls cholesterol and blood sugar levels. It also will keep your body young.

In addition, weight training's benefits continue long after you've hit the showers, says

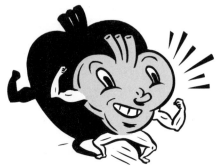

Chris Melby, Dr.P.H., director of the Human Energy Laboratory at Colorado State University in Fort Collins. Dr. Melby put 13 men through a rigorous 90-minute weight-lifting session. "The morning after intense resistive exercise, we found the metabolic rate elevated in all but one participant," he says. There also was some indication that their rate of fat burning was elevated the morning after weight lifting compared to the morning before. In another study researchers found that older people who lifted weights three times a week burned an extra 100 calories a day, enough to stave off ten pounds of fat over a year.

Another study by researchers at the Oregon Health Sciences University in Portland found that after a 16-week program where 30 middle-age men either jogged, lifted weights or did nothing, the runners and weight lifters decreased body fat. But only the weight lifters increased their lean body mass—more commonly known as muscle. The runners, as you'd expect, increased their lung capacities more.

We're not saying you should rely on weight lifting to exercise your heart and lungs, or to get the general health benefits once considered the sole realm of aerobic exercise. Rather, by combining resistance and aerobic training, you can greatly enhance your strength, stamina and health in more ways than once believed.

Aiming for the Heart

To have a stronger, better heart, you need to be in the zone—the target training zone, the heart rate that promotes the best possible cardiovascular fitness. Exercise experts say that zone is between 70 to 85 percent of your maximum heart rate. Instead of doing a lot of math, find your zone on this handy chart.

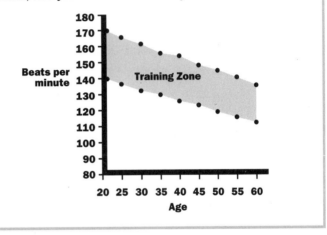

A Hearty Workout

Here's how to improve cardiovascular fitness both in and out of the gym.

Get a health screening. Your first step is to get a checkup, says Laura A. Gladwin, a fitness consultant, lecturer and owner of L.G.A. Fitness Consulting and Training in Brea, California. "You need to know where you stand health-wise before you jump into an exercise program," she says, adding that you should also get an evaluation of body composition, flexibility, aerobic fitness (VO_2 max, which measures how efficiently your body uses oxygen) and muscular strength and endurance.

Hoof it. "Guys may not think it's macho to walk, but walking is probably the most highly prescribed form of fitness today," Gladwin says. So take some time each day to hoof it in the hallways, up the stairs, to the health club or to the grocery store. Walk around between sets during your workout.

Alternate days. If you don't have the time to squeeze aerobic training into your weight-lifting schedule, designate separate days for each. Yes, it'll take more time, but it'll also make you healthier—and give you the endurance to lift longer in future sessions.

"A lot of people become a little one-sided in their exercise programs, but you can't neglect the other side of the coin," says Steve J. Fleck, Ph.D., a sports physiologist in the Sports Science and Technology Division of the U.S. Olympic Committee in Colorado Springs, Colorado.

Your Body Type

Making Your Genes Fit

For poker players "luck of the draw" has a ring of finality to it. You can discard once and hope that your hand will improve—then you're stuck. In real life you're dealt a body with certain genetic characteristics. But unlike poker, you get to upgrade your hand as much as you please, and no one calls it cheating. In other words, you don't have to settle for hand-me-down genes.

"We inherit a certain amount of our body type from our parents, and that genetic constitution has a big impact on our body weight, our height and our percentage of body fat," says Colorado State University's Dr. Chris Melby. "But in addition to that, we have the behavioral factors that interact with our genetic constitution—what we eat, how much we eat and how much we exercise or don't exercise."

The idea is not to get obsessed with looking like one of those rippling hunks in the underwear ads. It would be much more productive to check out your *own* body's characteristics and develop a reasonable, tailor-made training program.

"I get irritated with Madison Avenue and the fashion magazines that suggest people all need to look very lean when in fact they may not be genetically set up to be that way," says Dr. Melby. "They're told they don't have much value unless they are. And that's really a travesty."

Mighty Morphin' Power

Fitness professionals recognize three basic body shapes:

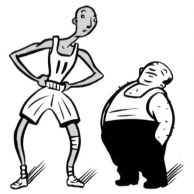

endomorphs (round), mesomorphs (muscular) and ectomorphs (lean).

Dutch researchers, for instance, put 21 sedentary men through a weight-training program of 14 exercises twice a week for 12 weeks. Ten of the men were slender, and 11 were solidly built. The two groups showed comparable strength gains and fat loss during the training. But while the solidly built group showed considerable muscle buildup, the slender group showed none—even though their strength had increased equally. The scientists theorized that the two groups were genetically different, either in their potential to build muscle or in the speed at which their bodies adapt to training.

A massive, ongoing research project at Arizona State University in Tempe, involving five colleges and 650 subjects, indicates that 5 to 10 percent of people who work out are destined to show only modest gains. Most of the research subjects show moderate improvement in training programs, and another 5 to 10 percent are those fortunate souls who respond like genies released from a bottle. Part of the reason for these differences: Performance factors such as maximum oxygen uptake, lung capacity, muscle fiber and body type are influenced by genetics.

A man's body shape, by the way, is not a foolproof indication of his health or fitness level. "A person's outward appearance doesn't necessarily match his 'inward appearance,' his body composition," notes Dr. Wayne W. Campbell of the Noll Physiological Research Center at Pennsylvania State University.

"You could be an extremely fit-looking person and still have a low amount of muscle and a high amount of fat if you carry it well. On the other hand, you can be very not-fit-looking or pudgy, yet really be solid and mostly muscle," Dr. Campbell says.

Custom Bodywork

All three body types—endomorphs, mesomorphs and ectomorphs—can be improved with diet and exercise. Here are training strategies for each.

Endomorphs

These are the Babe Ruths of the world, large-framed and relatively high in body fat. They may or may not be well-muscled. Endomorphs are naturals at powering through moderately intense, long-haul activities such as cycling, Alpine skiing, rowing and football.

Disadvantages: Their metabolisms often are slow, meaning they have to watch what they eat. They're also more vulnerable to heart disease and injury to the knees and ankles.

Training tip: Follow a low-fat diet, about 70 percent carbohydrate, 10 percent protein and 20 percent fat. Burn calories with moderate aerobic exercise. Also, tone and build muscle with weight training.

Mesomorphs

The Carl Lewis types are medium-framed and naturally well-muscled. They respond best to strength training and don't have to work overly hard to stay in shape.

Disadvantages: They're vulnerable to weight gain if they don't eat carefully. Their considerable musculature makes them a tad weighty for long-distance running and swimming.

Training tip: Go for a low-fat, high-carbohydrate diet: 60 percent carbohydrate, 15 percent protein and 25 percent fat. Split your workouts evenly between aerobics and strength training.

If the Shoe Fits . . .

Babe Ruth knew where his strengths lay, and it wasn't marathon running. Here's a list of activities that are best suited to specific body types. Maybe you're a champion in search of the right sport.

Endomorph	Mesomorph	Ectomorph
Walking	Sprinting	Cycling
Cycling	Cycling	Basketball
Swimming	Football	Nordic skiing
Alpine skiing	Ice hockey	High jump
Baseball	Basketball	Pole vault
Ice hockey	Track events	Tennis
Rowing	Windsurfing	Volleyball
Football	Racquetball	Weight training
Basketball	All types of skiing	Long-distance running
	Weight training	
	Baseball	

Ectomorphs

Think of Kareem Abdul-Jabbar—light-framed, low in both fat and muscle. Ectomorphs are energetic, nimble and naturals at endurance. It doesn't take much of a workout for them to keep trim, and they're less prone to heart disease.

Disadvantages: They have to work harder to build muscle. Also, envious endomorphs and mesomorphs hope they'll choke on their Twinkies.

Training tip: Emphasize carbohydrates and moderate amounts of protein to keep those muscles primed and working. Aim for a diet that contains 65 percent carbohydrate, 15 percent protein and 20 percent fat. Work out with weights to build muscle, plus make sure you get light aerobic activity to keep the heart honest.

Age and Exercise

A Word to the Wizened: Grow Strong, Live Long

At age 45 George Foreman knocked out Michael Moorer and reclaimed the heavyweight boxing title he had lost 20 years earlier.

A month before he turned 38, weight lifter Norbert Schemansky snatched 164.2 kilograms for a world record.

And as he entered his fifth decade, Ashrita Furman held the record for holding records in the Guinness Book of World Records—ten number one spots, all of them for athletic pursuits such as somersaulting, deep knee bends and basketball dribbling.

So, how will biographers say you spent *your* middle age? Give me a break, you protest, those guys are all muscular mutants! The only physical phenomenon that normal guys can look forward to is a long, slow slide toward that black abyss. Right?

Wrong.

"There's nothing special about even world-class athletes. They're human beings just like we are," says Furman, the manager of a health food store in New York City. "At Jamaica High School I skipped gym class all the time. I was a wimp. It's funny, because now that's where I train. My phys ed teacher can't believe that it's the same guy 20 years later."

You may not plan to swim the English Channel in your forties or scale Mt. Everest on your 75th birthday, but you probably do share an ambition with every guy since Ponce de León: to stop, or at least slow, the aging process. You want to live long, well and independently, looking

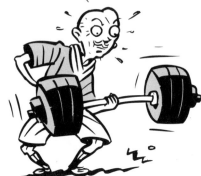

and feeling good. All of this, scientists say, you *can* achieve—by weight training.

The Aging of Aquarians

If you dread getting older, maybe that's because of what you see in the population around you. United States government health officials say that fewer than 15 percent of adults between the ages of 18 and 74 get regular vigorous exercise. The result is an epidemic of maladies related to long-term bodily neglect, such as heart disease, high blood pressure, diabetes, back problems, bone degeneration and debilitating muscular weakness. If that sums up your concept of aging, you'll be relieved to know that strength training can help counteract all of those health problems.

You've heard of the use-it-or-lose-it principle: Muscle that gets used stays put or enlarges; unused muscle shrinks. If you don't get off your duff, in other words, you can kiss your gluteus maximus good-bye.

A few years back, it seemed everyone in the country was making jokes about those obnoxious television commercials in which an elderly person cried, "I've fallen and I can't get up." But with the population getting older, muscular decline is a problem that doctors and scientists are taking more and more seriously. Falls already are the number one killer for people in their eighties, according to the National Safety Council. And U.S. citizens are in for more than a touch of gray in the coming decades. By the year 2001, baby boomers will just begin to slide into the age 55-plus category, and by the year 2030, nearly a third of the U.S. population will be 55 or older.

"From the time that you're in your forties or early fifties until you're in your seventies and eighties, you lose roughly 1 percent of your strength per year, or about 10 percent per decade," says Dr. Wayne W. Campbell of the Noll Physiological Research Center at Pennsylvania State University.

Getting Off Your Rocker

The physical advantages of weight training—increased muscle, better coordination and higher metabolism—are within the grasp of all adults, even those in their nineties.

"The studies that look at older people who are vigorously exercising show they can maintain a more 'youthful' bodily composition with exercise programs," says Dr. Campbell. "This suggests that a very large component of muscular decline is inactivity— not using your muscles enough for them to want to stick around."

In Boston, for instance, researchers studied 100 frail nursing home residents ranging in age from 72 to 98. They were put through intense hip and knee workouts—45-minute sessions, three times a week for ten weeks. The residents showed increases in muscle strength (113 percent), gait speed (11 percent) and stair-climbing power (28 percent). Four of those elderly exercisers surrendered their walkers by the end of the ten weeks and got by with canes.

Stanford University and Veterans Affairs researchers got 25 people ages 61 to 78 to weight-train for a year in Palo Alto, California. The subjects worked out for an hour three times a week, and their routines, which included three sets of 12 lifting exercises, covered all the major muscle groups. The exercisers got stronger rapidly during the first three months of the study and plateaued for the rest of the year. Some of the participants showed

You're No Slouch

Few things will add undeserved years to your appearance like bad posture. Walking tall will not only make you look younger, but it will help ward off back pain and give you more power in sports. Further, because you breathe better upright, you'll get more oxygen and have more energy.

First, you have to learn how to walk: Tighten your belly muscles, keep your butt tucked in, pull in your chin and don't lock your knees.

Next, strengthen your back, abdominal and butt muscles. This exercise gives them all a workout: Lie face down on the floor, arms bent at the elbows, palms and forearms on the floor, like a Sphinx. Slowly lift your head and chest up as far as you can comfortably go, keeping your palms and forearms on the floor. Then slowly let yourself down again. When you can do this easily ten times, try it with your arms at your sides. The next level: hands under your chin and elbows out. Superman level: arms extended forward, keeping an eye out for Kryptonite.

strength gains of more than 90 percent in their hip and leg muscles.

Scientists also believe strength training can help fend off some crippling diseases. In one study elderly exercisers lost none of their bone content over six months, while their counterparts who did not exercise lost 2 percent. In another study researchers reviewed the activity levels of 6,815 Japanese American men between the ages of 45 and 68 in the Honolulu Heart Program. They concluded that the most active guys—those in the top 20 percent, who were accustomed to lifting, shoveling, carpentry and the like—had cut their risk of diabetes in half.

Are You Fit?

Put Yourself to the Test

Competition. It's just part of being male, right? Inherent in the Y chromosome? Seems like we're always whipping out that mental measuring tape to compare ourselves to other guys—who caught the biggest fish, has the fastest car or makes the most money.

Sizing yourself up physically, though, is not just an exercise in envy. It tells you how well you're combating the aging process and how you need to fine-tune your training program.

What follows is a simple series of tests to point you in the right direction. It's nothing like a thorough physical checkup—you still have to pay your doctor for that. And proceed with care. If you are unaccustomed to physical exertion, have high blood pressure, have had chest pain, have heart trouble in your family or are 20 pounds overweight, you'd better give your doc a call first.

Strength

You could always have a forger change the date of birth on your driver's license. But that would do nothing to combat the muscular decline that comes with aging. The average guy loses a half pound of muscle every year between the ages of 20 and 50. With strength training you get the *body* of a younger man, not just the I.D. of one.

According to Wayne Westcott, Ph.D., strength-training consultant to the YMCA and other national organizations, the following are a couple of tests to check out your upper- and lower-body strength.

Chair lift. According to Dr. Westcott, this test gauges upper-body strength. Sit on the edge of an exercise bench or a stable, armless chair. Stick your legs straight out, heels on the floor and toes pointing up. Plant a hand on either side of the bench or chair for support and slide your bottom off the edge. Now touch your butt to the floor, pause one second and push back up. If you're a moderately strong guy in your twenties, you should be able to do ten chair lifts. If you're older, subtract one from that goal for every extra decade. (In your thirties, it's nine lifts, and so on.)

One-minute squat. This slow-motion squat is a test of both power and endurance in your lower body, says Dr. Westcott. The goal is to take 30 seconds lowering yourself and 30 seconds rising. Stand and spread your feet to shoulder width. Very slowly, bend your knees until your hips are just below your knees. Keep your heels on the floor. Then very slowly raise yourself back up. If you're in your twenties, you should be able to handle the full minute. In your thirties, 50 to 55 seconds; in your forties, 45 to 50 seconds; in your fifties, 40 to 45 seconds; sixties and up, 40 seconds or less.

Body Fat

If love handles ever got used the way their name implies, you might think twice about getting rid of them. That not being the case, however, you're better off torching any excess flab with a combination of exercise and diet.

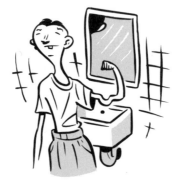

According to Dr. Westcott, the following skinfold test will show how you stack up—or stick out—in the fat department. Ask a friend to do the measuring. It's tough to get an accurate measurement by yourself, and asking a random stranger might get you in trouble.

Skinfold test. Hold your arm straight out in front of

1.5 Mile Run Test

This test from The Cooper Institute for Aerobics Research in Dallas is intended for healthy people who are already active. If you are sedentary, try a walking program for several weeks before you try this, and if you are ill or have symptoms such as chest pain, check with your doctor before you attempt the 1.5 mile run.

Find a track and mark off 1.5 miles, or on a 440-yard track, 1.5 miles equals six laps running in the inside lane.

Don't push yourself to complete exhaustion—work at or just beyond the higher intensities of your current workout program. Practice pacing yourself so you don't exhaust yourself before you finish the test.

Don't eat for two hours before running, and warm up and stretch. Afterward cool down for five minutes.

Check your time to find out how you did.

	Twenties	Thirties	Forties	Fifties	Sixties
Superior	faster than 8:13	faster than 8:44	faster than 9:30	faster than 10:40	faster than 11:20
Excellent	8:14–10:16	8:45–10:47	9:31–11:44	10:41–12:51	11:21–13:53
Good	10:17–11:41	10:48–12:20	11:45–13:14	12:52–14:24	13:54–15:29
Fair	11:42–12:51	12:21–13:36	13:15–14:29	14:25–15:26	15:30–16:43
Poor	12:52–14:13	13:37–14:52	14:30–15:41	15:27–16:43	16:44–18:00
Very poor	slower than 14:13	slower than 14:52	slower than 15:41	slower than 16:43	slower than 18:00

you, with your palm up. Use your thumb and forefinger to grasp the skin on the underside of your forearm. Don't squeeze tightly, and be sure not to pinch any muscle. Have a friend measure the distance between your finger and thumb with a ruler. If you're between ages 20 and 40, three-fourths of an inch is average and one-half of an inch is good. For guys ages 40 to 60, seven-eighths of an inch is average and five-eighths of an inch is good.

Flexibility

"Bend, but don't break" works for aspens and athletes alike. Training for flexibility will go a long way toward preventing muscle pulls and tears while performing any physical activity. Dr. Westcott suggests the following test as a way to evaluate how much reach you're getting out of your back and legs.

Toe touch. Sit on the floor in the figure 4 position: left leg straight out, heel of your right foot against your left thigh. Reach with your left hand toward your toes. If you're between the ages of 20 and 40, being able to touch your wrist to your toe is good; fingertips to toe, average; fingers to ankle, fair; fingers to sockline, poor. Guys ages 40 to 60 get a slight break: Fingertips to toe rates a "good," and so on.

Eating for Power

Fueling Your Muscle Machine

You're not the same man you were six months ago. No, it's not the new sport coat. It's not the new magazine you subscribed to. And it's not your new forehand grip.

Literally, the meat on your bones is not the same beef that was hanging there half a year ago. Your body is constantly replenishing itself, and it takes only six months to scrap and rebuild every muscle fiber in your body. In a year's time even your bones are shown the door and replaced.

Where does all this building material come from? The food you eat. So if you have a steady diet of burgers and fries, you'll get a larded, burger-and-fries kind of body. If you go the Food Guide Pyramid route—meaning you eat a wide range of foods and emphasize whole grains, pasta, fruits and vegetables—you'll wind up with a rock-solid bod and plenty of energy to move it around.

"The bottom line is to meet your metabolic needs and to be able to stick with that," says Baltimore physical therapist and trainer Bob Viau. "Athletes train themselves to view food much differently: as fuel for the body. The result is a much different body type and a different attitude toward eating."

Get a Carb Tune-Up

For most guys, shifting to a more powerful diet is a matter of fine-tuning rather than a total overhaul. The average man's diet is 35 percent fat, 45 percent carbohydrate and 20 percent protein. That protein level is good—keep it right there. But whittle the fat figure down to

20 percent and boost the carbohydrates to 60 percent. Now you're a lean, powerful machine.

Those carbohydrates are high-test gasoline for the body. During exercise your muscles are powered by a substance called glycogen, which your body makes from carbohydrates. Carbohydrates come from plant foods like potatoes, corn, rice, bananas, whole-wheat bread and pasta.

Yes, your muscles can burn fat as fuel, too, but it's metabolized much less efficiently. Research has shown that high-performance athletes can power themselves with fat. That means if you're the kind of guy who bike races through the Rocky Mountains all day for fun, you can get some mileage out of an extra cheeseburger without it padding your rear end. But for the everyday guy just trying to give his all to a bench press, bran flakes will fuel the job better than a burger any day.

Some researchers hinted that pasta—that beloved high-carb staple of endurance athletes—will actually make you fat. At issue was whether pasta could exacerbate a problem in some people called insulin resistance, causing carbohydrates to get converted into blubber under the belt. As yet, not many nutritionists are buying the theory, and they still lean toward linguine as a source of ready energy.

Here are more ways to put a little hop into your step throughout the day.

Manage your meals. If you want all-day energy, the best time to stoke your personal furnace is first thing in the morning. "Start with a

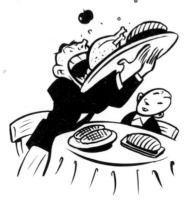

good breakfast. For most active individuals it should supply one-fourth to one-third of your daily calories," says Dr. Chris Melby of the Human Energy Laboratory at Colorado State University. Good bets are pancakes, cereal, fruit, juice, omelettes and muffins.

When energy reserves dip, you can feel irritable, headachy and ravenous. Snacks will help, but you have to choose the right foods. Bananas, bagels, fig bars and other foods high in complex carbohydrates will ensure a steady flow of fuel to your body.

Have a power lunch. Break up your day with exercise—it will energize you rather than make you tired. "I prefer to exercise at noon," Dr. Melby says. "There's a tendency for a lot of people in the middle of the afternoon to feel tired and not quite as productive. If I exercise fairly strenuously over the lunch hour and have a modest lunch, then I tend to have plenty of energy throughout the day."

Don't be late for dinner. The purpose of dinner is to power your evening's activities, and some doctors say it should be the lightest meal of the day. If you eat late—say, after 9:00 P.M.—those calories are less likely to be burned and more likely to be stored as fat.

Drink up. When you're working out, drink *before* you get thirsty. Otherwise, you run the risk of dehydration.

Plan ahead. If you're just planning a moderate workout, don't take in any calories in the previous hour. The digestion can sap energy from the muscles you want to exercise.

Many endurance athletes facing a big-time training session or race, however, like to pack in the carbohydrates over the preceding days and then guzzle a high-carbohydrate sports drink just before the event. One study examined runners who ran for 35 kilometers and then were asked to go all-out for another 5 kilometers. Those who'd had a high-carbohydrate sports drink just before the run maintained their pace longer and more powerfully than those who'd had nothing.

Sports drinks may not help with every activity, though. Twelve experienced tennis

---

Supplements: Who Needs 'Em?

Anyone who has set foot in a weight room has heard the suggestions: Gobble steak, scarf eggs, gulp supplements like protein powders and shakes.

Yes, your body does require protein to build muscle. But the average American male already consumes all the protein he needs in order to beef up. Your body needs about 35 grams of protein a day for basic functioning. To perform the incredible task of building a pound of muscle in a week, you would have to consume just 16 grams more a day, or 51 grams total. But most guys eat more than 100 grams of protein a day.

"The main thing with nutrition is to stay away from the supplements and have a healthy, balanced meal," says B. Don Franks, Ph.D., professor and chairman of the Department of Kinesiology at Louisiana State University in Baton Rouge. "There's no such thing as good and bad foods. The portions and the balance are what's important. Eat from all the food groups, get a lot of fruits and vegetables and limit the amount of fat and red meat. You don't need supplements even when you're training—vitamins, calcium, chromium and whatever else."

When you hear hype about athletes benefiting from protein and other supplements, check the supporting evidence. Chances are they're talking about high-performance pros who work out intensely a minimum of three hours a day. Is that you?

---

players were put through two three-hour matches, once with a high-carbohydrate sports drink to sip and another time with flavored, colored water. The sports drink offered no advantage in either playing ability or in maintaining fluid levels.

Flexing and Flexibility

Stretch Your Limbs— Not Your Luck

Remember the manager of your high school basketball team? He didn't have that star quality on the court, but without him the team machine would grind painfully to a halt.

Muscular flexibility is like that. Strength and endurance get all the glory. You want to hoist hundreds of pounds like those Olympians on TV or cycle up mountains without breaking a sweat. Flexibility doesn't get much airtime.

But it keeps you in the game. Flexibility provides better physical performance by giving you full use of your limbs, preventing debilitating injuries and making you look better by improving your posture.

"Flexibility is one of the key components of a balanced fitness program. When you're talking balanced fitness, you're talking strength training, cardiovascular training and flexibility training," says Ed Burke, Ph.D., associate professor at the University of Colorado at Colorado Springs and vice-president of the National Strength and Conditioning Association.

Flexibility is simply the ability to get a full range of motion out of a joint. If you can no longer serve tennis balls or turn in the driver's seat to glance behind you satisfactorily, you could have a flexibility problem.

The improved range of motion that comes with flexibility gives you an edge with your weight-lifting regimen, Dr. Burke says. Using proper range of motion during lifting exercises builds muscles evenly and thoroughly.

And speaking of strength training, forget the old-time notion that more muscle means less flexibility. "There is absolutely no evidence that strength gains come at the expense of flexibility," says Dr. Wade A. Lillegard of the Uniformed Services University of the Health Sciences. "You can have a bodybuilder or power lifter who's just as flexible as a dancer if they include stretching as part of their exercise routine."

A Joint Approach

The motion of a joint is affected by three things: the shape of the bones that meet in the joint, the surrounding ligaments and the elasticity of the tendons and muscles involved. That last factor is one you can control: You make a joint flexible by regularly stretching the muscles and tendons surrounding it.

Muscles that are not stretched frequently become shorter and tighter—particularly muscles that are kept strong through regular activity. Stretching is thought to lengthen small parts of the muscle fiber called sarcomeres. When your muscle is first stretched, your nerves get, well, nervous. They send messages to the muscle, telling it to contract to protect it from overstretching. When you hold the stretch for 20 seconds or more, the nerve impulses fade and allow a more thorough, more comfortable stretch.

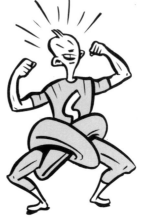

Stretching routines are usually simple. They should be part of any strength- or endurance-training program, but they also can be done separately or as part of a relaxation program such as tai chi or yoga.

Stretch for Success

"Stretching is very important before a workout so you don't go into it with really tight, cold muscles," says Dr. Wayne W. Campbell of the Noll Physiological Research Center at Pennsylvania State University. "It's equally important to do stretching after a workout so that your body's had a chance to relax while it's still doing things, as opposed to just abruptly stopping it."

Dr. Lillegard offers these guidelines for stretching.

Warm up. To work out safely, you need to first prime your body, says Dr. Lillegard. Do five or ten minutes of light aerobic exercise to get the blood moving and the muscles warm. Stretch, then work out. Cool down for five or ten more minutes with light activity and more stretches. This method will help prevent pulled muscles and reduce muscle and joint soreness.

Stretch slowly. Ease the joint to the limit of its movement, until you feel resistance but not any pain.

Don't be a jerk. Never stretch with a jerking or twisting motion. You can injure yourself that way.

Hold that stretch. Fitness experts generally recommend holding a stretch for 20 seconds or more. In fact, researchers at the University of Central Arkansas in Conway found that a 30-second stretch was ideal for improving hamstring flexibility. They divided 57 people into groups and assigned them to do stretches five days a week for six weeks. One group stretched for 15 seconds, another for 30 seconds and the third for 60 seconds. The people who stretched for 30 seconds acquired substantially more flexibility than those who stretched for 15 seconds. Those who stretched for 60 seconds improved no more than the 30-second bunch.

Build up slowly. If you're just starting out, you might need to gradually increase your stretching time. Try each stretch briefly four times with short rest periods in between. Do them daily, including weekends. It may take months before you notice any improvement.

Are You Flexible?

Here are some easy ways to test your flexibility. If you have back, hip or hamstring problems, check with your doctor before proceeding.

Hamstrings. Lie on your back with your butt against a wall and your legs extended up. Your knees should be bent, with your heels against the wall.

Slide your heels up the wall as you slowly straighten your knees. Don't force the stretch. Move your butt away from the wall a few inches until you can find a position that you can hold for 30 or more seconds. If you can straighten your knees comfortably without moving your rear away from the wall, your hamstrings are flexible. If you had to move your rear more than two inches away from the wall, they aren't.

Shoulders. Raise one arm like you're asking a question in class. Bend that elbow and reach down your back. Put the back of your other hand against your middle back and move it up. If your fingers meet, your shoulder is flexible. Switch sides and repeat.

Hips. Find a sturdy, knee-high surface, like a weight-room bench. With your feet flat on the floor, lie back on the bench, thighs parallel to the floor. Pull one knee up to your chest. If you can comfortably keep the other foot flat on the floor, your hip is flexible. Switch legs to test the other side.

Achieving Power

How to Be a He-Man for All Seasons

You want to be built like Bruce Willis, just in case a *Die Hard* kind of day comes along. Total, all-around power means having a body primed to tackle any physical task.

This requires total-body training. And that full spectrum of training includes not only working out the major muscle groups, but also aerobic exercise and training specific to your favorite sport. Flexibility and nutrition are essential as well. These elements are inextricably linked: Ignore any one and, as a superhero, you'll have trouble living through the opening credits.

Dr. Chris Melby of the Human Energy Laboratory at Colorado State University advocates swapping off between aerobic and weight-training workouts. "I typically encourage people to exercise about five times a week and to alternate between resistive and aerobic exercise," he says. "Maybe one week they will do aerobic exercise twice and strength training three times, and the next week they will do strength training twice and aerobic exercise three times. Alternating between different modes of exercise provides a good balance."

When you put strength training and aerobic training together, you get a powerful combination of fitness benefits. Both burn fat, aerobics by directly burning calories and weight lifting by raising the metabolism long-term. Weight lifting also helps you control blood sugar and strengthens the heart and bones, and may help lower and regulate blood pressure.

Maybe you've heard locker room talk that aerobic

and strength programs interfere with each other if they're carried out simultaneously. Scientists at the University of Wisconsin-Madison debunked that notion. They found 30 guys who hadn't exercised for at least three months and had them work out for ten weeks, three times a week. Ten of the men did strength training (eight exercises, four sets each), ten did endurance training (50 minutes of cycling) and ten did both workouts back-to-back on the same day. At the end of the study, the guys with the combined program made the same strength gains as the strength-only exercisers *and* they made the same aerobic gains as the aerobics-only exercisers. In short, they don't conflict. They complement each other.

Muscle: Why Bigger Is Better

When you lift weights, your body adapts to that level of exertion. The muscles grow. Then, you up the ante: more weight. Your muscles counter with more growth. In a sensible weight-training program you can expect to increase your strength by 5 percent per week, at the same time adding ½ pound of muscle to your body. This gives you a heck of an edge over the average guy, who loses ½ pound of muscle every year between the ages of 20 and 50 and gains 1½ pounds of fat per year.

Not only is that added muscle crucial to your fitness and lifestyle, but it also makes it easier to keep your body trim. For every pound of muscle you gain, your resting metabolic rate goes up 50 calories a day, meaning you can burn that much extra energy even if you're just lolling in the hammock.

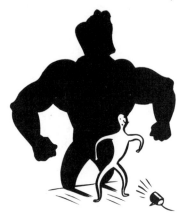

"Aerobic activity only burns calories while you're doing the activity and for a little while after," says Carlos DeJesus, a world-champion bodybuilder and fitness trainer in Richmond, Virginia. "But if you enlarge your muscles, now you're burning calories around the clock, because that bigger engine needs more fuel to work. So the idea is to go ahead and get those muscles as large as you can. I combine resistance training with aerobic conditioning to give my clients the best of both worlds."

The Path to Power

You don't want to waste any time or energy on inefficient exercise. For the best muscle-building effect, fitness experts recommend weight lifting two or three times a week, with at least a day's rest between sessions. Lift the most weight you can handle in the 8- to 12-rep range. A set like that should take you 1 to 1½ minutes to complete. At that level of exertion, the muscle will actually break down, heal and come back stronger than before—the essence of muscle-building. The heavier weight accelerates this process. (Lighter weights lifted at higher repetitions will primarily build endurance, not strength, fitness experts say.)

Now, here's where you need to examine your goals: If you're lifting weights to reap basic health benefits, then hitting all of the major muscle groups with one set each will do nicely. But if you're trying to raise your hulk quotient, do two or three sets at a time before moving on to the next exercise, with a minute or so of rest between sets. Scientists say that's the route to the quickest gains.

Remember that the weight room is not just a smorgasbord of cast iron where you can dive in and start lifting willy-nilly. For one thing, researchers say you'll get the most muscle growth if you begin with the large muscle groups (chest, shoulders, legs, back, abdominals) and work your way down to the smaller muscles such as the triceps and biceps. Suppose you did the opposite—you fatigued

Weights and Weight Loss

Overweight people often avoid strength training for fear they'll gain weight, not lose it. That's unfortunate, because when you cut calories without exercise, you can lose muscle as well as fat.

Dr. Wayne Westcott, strength-training consultant to the YMCA and other national organizations, studied 313 people who combined a low-fat diet with a program of strength training and aerobic exercise. After eight weeks they had lost eight pounds of fat and gained three pounds of muscle. The scales may have only recorded a net weight loss of five pounds, but that doesn't begin to tell the whole story. Lean muscle mass burns calories at a revved-up rate—during rest as well as during exercise. So the three added pounds of muscle served as a 24-hour-a-day fat furnace.

the triceps with a push-down exercise first, and then you did a bench press, which also calls on the triceps. Your bench press will be less effective because your triceps are pooped, and your entire chest will get less benefit from the lift.

Balance is important, too. You'll find that muscles are generally balanced on either side of a joint: biceps versus triceps, quadriceps versus hamstrings, and chest versus upper back. Strengthening muscle on one side of a joint while neglecting the other side can lead to injury. So don't play favorites.

Last Longer and Stronger

You want to win five-set tennis matches and still go dancing that night. You want to spend hours whispering through a snow-blanketed forest on cross-country skis. You want to haul your backpack up and down mountains all day, then bounce out of your sleeping bag raring to do it again the next morning.

This is where you rely on your endurance training, which improves the performance of your heart, lungs and metabolism. The traditional aerobic activities—like running, cycling, swimming, hiking and rowing—all build endurance.

Endurance programs vary greatly depending on individual preferences and goals. But they do share a general approach: small, gradual improvements in the training program. "It's hard to make people understand this," says Dr. B. Don Franks of the Department of Kinesiology at Louisiana State University. "But if they're going to do it safely, they have to take a gradual approach, where they don't have the pain and discomfort that people associate with basic training. There's no need for that."

Working Your Way Up

Say you want to start a running program to complement your strength training, but you get winded after several minutes on the track. "You can try a kind of interval program where you walk, then you jog a while, you walk, you jog a while, and you're being guided mainly by comfort," Dr. Franks says. "When you feel any kind of discomfort, then you go back to a walk. When you get rested, you can jog again. And you gradually jog more."

Once you're able to jog for 3 miles every other day, says Dr. Franks, you've reached an important benchmark: You're probably ready for vigorous endurance sports like racquetball, tennis or high-impact aerobics. The equivalent milestone for walkers is 6 miles; for bicyclists, 12 miles; and for swimmers, ¾ of a mile.

High-performance endurance athletes—

How to Get Started

We asked a panel of experts some of the most common questions weight lifters encounter. Here's what they said.

How often should I lift? Your schedule dictates how much time you spend in the gym. Start with two days a week and progress to three. For maximum muscle-building, work four days a week. Just rest each muscle group at least 24 hours after a workout so it can rebuild—and grow.

How many reps should I do? View repetitions as a scale of 1 to 25. One represents maximum power, 25 maximum endurance. The 1-rep approach is what an Olympic power lifter does. Average lifters seeking power won't be so extreme; they'll stick to 3 to 5 reps. Eight to 12 reps are better for mainstream bodybuilding. Working in that range gives you muscular growth and definition. Fifteen reps and beyond won't build much muscle, but it will tone and build muscular endurance.

How many sets should I do? Two sets per muscle group is a fine starting point for most guys. Then work your way up to three sets per muscle group. If you've done that and want faster growth, consider multiple sets for each muscle group. For example, to build your chest pronto, you'd do bench presses and dumbbell flies in the same workout instead of one or the other.

How much weight should I use? To start, find a weight that you can lift comfortably and then do your reps with slightly less. Lifting too much to start can cause poor

marathoners and triathletes, for instance—need to train four to six times a week, fitness experts say. But at that pace, stress injuries become a concern for runners, who may want to incorporate into their routines lower-impact exercises

Warm Up and Cool Down

The owner's manual of your car probably warns you not to start it up cold and immediately roar down the highway at 65 miles per hour. You need to drive moderately for a few minutes, allowing the car's innards to warm up before they're ready for high performance. The same goes for your body. According to Dr. Franks, before any intense endurance exercise you need to do two things: warm up and stretch. This can reduce soreness, keep you flexible and prevent injury.

If you're moderately fit, he says five or ten minutes of very light exercise will raise your heart rate and prime your circulatory system, lungs and muscles for exercise. Walking does this well. Or try an easy-going version of the workout you're preparing for. If you're bicycling, pedal around slowly for a few minutes. If you're playing handball, jog easily around the court first while you give the ball a few friendly practice swats.

Now you're ready for stretches, which ensure that your body parts can glide safely through the full range of motion. Remember that stretching is not a vigorous activity—quick or bouncing movements can injure your muscles.

To cool down after exercise, do the same five or ten minutes of walking and stretching. "If you just stop immediately, it's dangerous," says Dr. Franks. "You still have the need for extra blood after the work that you've done, but it pools in the legs if you stop, and it's not getting pumped back to the heart. So some light activity is very important to do afterwards."

Continue your cooldown activity until you feel nearly rested, you're not breathing hard and you're no longer sweating.

technique or injury. Once you're comfortable with the lighter weight and proper technique, increase the resistance for your next workout by adding just five to ten pounds at a clip. The goal is to feel thoroughly fatigued on your last set.

How fast should I lift the weights? Weight lifting is not a race. If you're lifting light weights for endurance, you can quickly—and safely—power through your reps as long as you keep good form and technique. Same for power lifting, where you need only one burst of maximum power. Otherwise, lift your weight in two seconds and lower it in four. This helps maintain proper rhythm and technique.

How long should I rest between sets? For heavy lifting—say, 85 to 90 percent of your one-repetition maximum (the most you can lift in one burst)—wait two to three minutes between sets. For moderate lifting—70 to 80 percent of your repetition maximum—wait a minute or less. For light lifting—40 to 60 percent of your repetition maximum—30 seconds or less will do.

Our experts: Ed Burke, Ph.D., associate professor at the University of Colorado at Colorado Springs and vice-president of the National Strength and Conditioning Association; Steve J. Fleck, Ph.D., sports physiologist in the Sports Science and Technology Division of the U.S. Olympic Committee in Colorado Springs, Colorado; James E. Graves, Ph.D., associate professor and chair of the Department of Health and Education at Syracuse University in New York; Peter Lemon, Ph.D., professor of applied physiology at Kent State University in Kent, Ohio; Harvey Newton, instructor at the University of Colorado at Colorado Springs and director of program development for the National Strength and Conditioning Association.

like swimming, bicycling or running in place in deep water. Also, you need to calculate in how you add time and intensity to an endurance workout. Be sure to peak just in time for that big competition.

Injury-Free Power

How to Gain Muscle without Pain

Before you enter a weight room, banish any thoughts of heroics and showmanship. You might be thinking Schwarzenegger, but the only thing you'll terminate by piling on too much weight is your ability to work out.

"People tend to go into a gym, see a guy doing heavy resistance work, and say, 'I'm gonna do *that!*' And that's where folks get into trouble," says David H. Janda, M.D., an orthopedic surgeon and director of the Institute for Preventive Sports Medicine in Ann Arbor, Michigan.

Training on free weights or machines is generally safe if you know what you're doing. One study of almost 11,000 college football players showed that only 34 players were injured in weight rooms over a four-year period that included 297,000 training sessions. But remember that college athletes have loads of input from coaches, trainers and teammates to help prevent accidents. If accidents can still happen with such an elaborate support system, you'd better bone up on safety before you wrap your hands around your first dumbbell.

Practice Safe Flex

Studying adolescent and young adult weight lifters, researchers from the University of Texas in Houston concluded that the greatest risk of technique-related weight room injury came during aggressive use of free weights, in exercises such as the deadlift and the bench press. While

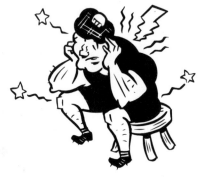

machines are considered safer than free weights, particularly for beginners, they aren't fool-proof, either.

Our experts offer these guidelines for safe strength training.

Check with Doc. Get your doctor to check you out before you start a strength-training program. You might have to modify or avoid weight lifting if you have muscle or joint problems, seizure disorders, heart disease, high blood pressure, previous injuries or other medical conditions, says Dr. Wade A. Lillegard of the Uniformed Services University of the Health Sciences.

Warm up. A warm-up reduces your risk of injury by increasing your blood flow and prepping your muscles for the work they're about to do, says fitness trainer Carlos DeJesus. Get a light aerobic workout first, using all the muscles you are going to work, by doing an activity such as jogging or cycling for five or ten minutes. Then stretch, holding the stretch on your large muscles for 30 seconds, and on your smaller muscles for 20 seconds. Don't bounce. Next perform a warm-up version of the weight lifting planned for that session, using very light weights and high repetitions. More light activity and stretching are recommended after the workout as a cooldown.

Study technique. Using the proper lifting form is important not only to work your muscles correctly, but also to prevent injury. Do your exercise through the full range of motion in a slow, controlled way.

Learn how to breathe. Normally, if you have to think about breathing, you're in trouble. But proper breathing technique is essential in weight lifting. If you hold your breath while pushing a heavy weight, you risk raising your blood pressure, Dr. Lillegard says. You should exhale during the main exertion and inhale during the relaxation phase.

Use a spotter. Most of

the serious weight-lifting accidents happen to people who are training with free weights by themselves. You particularly need a spotter when you are doing a bench press or squats near your weight limit, DeJesus says. Make sure your spotter keeps his mind on the job and is strong enough to get you out of a jam. Be sure you and your spotter have a plan, so that each of you knows exactly what the other will do in case you can't complete the lift.

Neatness counts. Don't leave equipment lying around the weight room where someone could trip over it. Always use the collars that prevent weights from falling off barbells.

Mind the machines. Keep your hands away from the chains, cams, pulleys and weight plates of exercise machines when they're in use, DeJesus cautions. When you select a weight, stick the key in all the way.

Pay Attention to Pain

Your body has a good alarm system. When a workout causes you pain, pay attention. Knowing how to react can help you avoid serious injury.

"I'm not a proponent of the 'no pain, no gain' theory," Dr. Janda says. In a weight-training program that emphasizes slow-and-steady progress, "you might feel the stretching of the muscle in your leg—that's different from out-and-out pain. But if you're working out and you say, 'Geez, this is really hurting,' you have to back off because you're probably causing injury more than you're causing good. It doesn't have to hurt in order for it to be good for you."

Fitness experts say exercise can cause several types of pain, including:
- *Pain during or just after a workout.* During a workout, repeated contractions cause substances such as lactic acid,

---

For Injuries, R.I.C.E. Is Nice

Just as Jerry Rice has set the standard for pro football receivers, the R.I.C.E. method is in a league of its own for treating sprains and muscle tears. According to Dr. David H. Janda, of the Institute for Preventive Sports Medicine, follow these steps to speed healing and reduce damage and swelling.

- *Rest.* When you're hurt, stop your workout immediately and take weight off the affected area.
- *Ice.* Wrap ice in a towel and hold it against the injury for 10 to 20 minutes, three or four times a day until the acute injury diminishes.
- *Compress.* Wrap the injured area in a snug, but not tight, elastic bandage.
- *Elevate.* Raise the injured limb and rest it on a pillow to reduce swelling.

---

other acids, proteins and hormones to build up in the muscle. This can cause pain even without injury. But if you experience a sharp, continuous pain, or pain accompanied by a burning sensation, stop lifting and get it checked by a doctor.
- *Delayed soreness.* Pain that appears a day or two after exercise is officially known as delayed onset muscle soreness (DOMS). "Eccentric" movements such as lowering a weight cause this kind of pain. To avoid DOMS, be sure to increase the weight you lift very gradually, so that your muscles can adapt comfortably.
- *Cramps.* These happen when muscles, often in the calves or feet, knot up in violent contractions. Cramps are most common in endurance sports like cycling and running when the athlete loses a lot of fluids through sweating. The best way to stop a cramp is to gently stretch the cramped muscle. Massage also might help.

Making Time

Get on Board the Fitness Express

In the time it took you to watch *Ernest Scared Stupid*, you could have done a week's worth of strength training and, probably, preserved a couple of IQ points.

Fitness experts generally recommend that you devote 20 to 30 minutes to strength training three times a week. Those sessions need to be separated by a day of rest, because weight-trained muscles need at least 48 hours to mend. That makes a Monday-Wednesday-Friday training pattern pretty popular.

If you're worried about that chock-full appointment calendar, muscle science actually works in your favor. The biggest strength gains are made when you lift the most weight you can handle for a relatively short period of time—one set of 8 to 12 reps—meaning that the most effective workouts also save time.

"Most people look for ways to make exercise easier. But you need to look for ways to make your exercise *harder*," says Ellington Darden, Ph.D., a fitness expert and strength-training researcher in Gainesville, Florida, and author of the book *Living Longer Stronger*. "Don't look for ways to do more exercise. Look for ways to do less, by efficiency. It takes very little time to get your body in shape, and even less to keep it there."

Twice Is Nice

If you're new to weight training, maybe working out three times a week sounds inhibiting. Take heart. A study conducted by the YMCA reported that out-of-shape subjects who exercised for just 20 minutes twice a week

built up an average of three extra pounds of muscle and shed more than four pounds of fat in less than eight weeks.

First, get a clear idea of what your goals are. At the very least, you can get some amount of health benefit just by keeping active.

"That can include carrying your groceries up the stairs versus taking the elevator or walking briskly three times a day for ten minutes," says Dr. Wayne W. Campbell of the Noll Physiological Research Center at Pennsylvania State University. "That's not going to get you fit. But it can give significant health benefits."

If your goal is true muscular fitness, says Dr. Campbell, "My minimum recommendation is weight lifting twice a week using the major muscle groups from your upper, middle and lower body. Focus on the large muscle groups—for example, the chest press or bench press, leg extensions, leg flexions, double leg presses, squat exercises, biceps curls, back exercises. That's a foundation for weight lifting."

Consider Convenience

Your workout itself might not be easy, but getting to your exercise equipment should be. If you have to drive 45 minutes to get to your gym, you'll start to view working out as a liability. Don't forget, though, that strength training can be done in a number of ways. Consider how those alternatives will mesh most efficiently with your lifestyle.

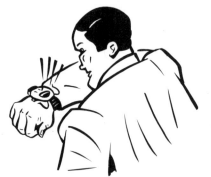

Machines are easy to use: You just push a metal pin into a stack of weights to choose the resistance level, then get lifting. Although free weights appear even simpler than machines, they require more attention to technique. But you don't necessarily have to join a club to get at them. If you spend more time on the road than in your own living room, the rubber tubing used for some resistance exercises can fold up inside a briefcase. And the one piece of exercise equipment you're never without is your own body, so calisthenics offer the ultimate strength-training convenience.

"Muscle doesn't care where it's getting its resistance—it's going to respond," says Dr. Wade A. Lillegard of the Uniformed Services University of the Health Sciences. "The resistance can be anything: body weight, rubber tubing, free weights, machines."

Here are more ways to get the most muscle out of the fewest minutes.

Get strength in numbers. Pick exercises that work several major muscle groups at the same time. The leg press, for example, targets the quadriceps, hamstrings, buttocks and calves. Essentially, you're doing four exercises simultaneously.

Speed it up. Skip the usual minute recovery time between exercises. You can do this by alternating upper- and lower-body exercises. Your upper-body muscles rest while the lower-body ones are being worked.

Lean toward machines. If you're pressed for time, do your bench presses—and other resistance exercises—on machines. There's nothing inherently wrong with barbells, but loading and unloading weight plates can burn up precious time. If you're pining for free weights, work in a couple of barbell exercises that you can perform one after the other without having to adjust the weight.

Call for backup. Every gym has at least one galoot who seems to set up permanent residence on a piece of equipment that's vital to your workout. You have no time to waste on bench hogs, so have a backup plan for each of your exercises: an alternate lift that hits the same muscle groups.

Make every minute count. The

---

20 Minutes to Muscle

For the man who doesn't have a millisecond to spare, here's how to get an all-around strength-training workout in just 20 minutes.

Do eight to ten repetitions of each exercise in the order listed. With just 15 seconds between exercises, your heart rate will stay elevated, providing some aerobic benefit, too. You should be able to work through the whole routine twice in 15 minutes, leaving time for warm-up and cooldown.

Here are two variations of the routine, one for gym equipment and the other for doing at home with just an exercise bench, a set of adjustable dumbbells and a chinning bar.

At the gym: Bench press, lat pull-down, military press, triceps pull-down, back extension.

At home: Dumbbell bench press (instead of alternating, do both sides at once), lunge with dumbbells, one-armed dumbbell bent-over row, dumbbell military press (do both sides at once), pull-up, seated triceps extension, concentration curl.

To do the seated triceps extension, sit on an exercise bench with your back straight and your feet on the floor. Grasp a single dumbbell in both hands. As you raise it over your head, tilt it until it's vertical and the top plate rests against your hands. This is the starting position. Lower by bending your elbows behind your head until your forearms touch your biceps. Raise the weight back to the starting position.

---

undisciplined exerciser allows lots of downtime to creep into his workout. Pack beneficial activity into every moment you're in the gym. Jogging in place, jumping jacks or stretches beat just standing around any day.

Secrets to Staying Motivated

Positive Outlook Breeds Positive Results

If it were strictly up to the rational part of your mind, you'd promptly file all receipts for the IRS in the same place. You'd quit playing poker with those barracudas at the corner bar. And you'd never butter another baked potato.

You also would hit the gym at least three times a week. You know the science, and it's inarguable: Exercise will make you look better, feel better and live longer. But you're flesh and blood, not an android. Your logic and your good intentions are forever getting mugged by a roving band of human foibles.

It's a phenomenon that worries fitness researchers. About half of the participants will typically drop out of a structured exercise program within six months. That drop-out rate, studies show, even applies to people who really ought to know better: cardiac patients. So when you start a training program, remember that hanging in there through the first several weeks is crucial. Your psyche is going to need major care and feeding.

One important motivation for exercise is the knowledge that you're doing the right thing. Considerable payoffs lie ahead, and a new you is emerging. People who exercise regularly list among their motivations not only improved health and fitness, but also better looks, social interaction, plain ol' fun and psychological benefits such as confidence, self-esteem and re-

lief from depression, anxiety and stress.

Hofstra University researchers in Hempstead, New York, studied 89 college students to determine the effects of exercise on mood. One group of students took a 90-minute swimming class twice a week for seven weeks, another group did weight lifting on the same schedule, and a third group sat on their duffs in an introductory psychology course. Both of the exercise groups showed a decline in depression by the end of the study. And the weight lifters alone got a bonus: substantially improved feelings about themselves.

"Some male clients come to me very withdrawn, very timid. They will start out wearing a sweatshirt, and the next thing I know they're wearing a T-shirt," says fitness trainer Carlos DeJesus. "By the time they start wearing a tank top they're there, whether they know it or not. They're feeling good about themselves, their pants have been pulled in three or four inches, they're strong, their shoulders are broader than their waist and they're in command. They're in control of themselves. They're doing new things: going into business, taking on a new sport or horseback riding, learning to play the piano. Their lives have become fuller."

Set Reasonable Goals

How do you bridge the gap between what you *do* and what you *should* do? First, master goal-setting. Goals focus your workout program and clarify what you're trying to achieve. As you attain each goal, you get that bounce of encouragement and cause for celebration.

Ashrita Furman, the holder of numerous number one spots in the Guinness Book of World Records, uses incremental goal-setting each

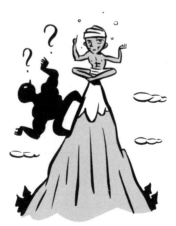

time he trains for a new sport. "I could only do 50 jumping jacks when I started," Furman says. "I would do 100 the next practice. Another practice I would do 200, another practice I would do 500. I'd get to 1,000, and then to the point where I could do 10,000 jumping jacks. The record at that time was 20,000 continuous jumping jacks. I did 27,000."

Here's how to ensure that the goals you set are not only achievable, but take you where you want to go.

Make your goals explicit. A vague goal, such as "I want to be strong," gives you nothing to shoot for. Instead say, "I'm going to lift weights three times a week until I can bench-press 150 pounds."

Be realistic. If you're an over-weight smoker, setting your sights on a marathon race will be an exercise all right—in frustration. First, see how far you can walk comfortably. Each time out, add a block or two to that distance until you're ready to mix in some jogging.

Reward yourself. What's the point of being victorious if you don't get some spoils now and then? For going a week without skipping a workout, treat yourself to your favorite ice cream.

Make It Fun

The surroundings are dingy, the equipment is medieval and the tasks are tedious. If that sounds like your workplace, let's hope you're paid well. If that sounds like your *workout*, then you won't get fired for making some changes. You're more likely to stick with a workout that's fun.

"I try to be well-rounded. I play basket-ball, I rollerblade with my kids, I play tennis, I

Excise Those Exercise Excuses

Now that you're brimming with positive thoughts, you're going to need a Dumpster for some of your old stumbling blocks—your favorite reasons for not exercising. Ready to heave-ho?

• *No time.* This was the excuse given by two-thirds of the "less active" people surveyed by the President's Council on Physical Fitness and Sports. But the same folks found at least three hours a week to watch TV. Chances are you also manage to read, go to movies and visit the pub occasionally. You do those things because they're fun and gratifying. With the right approach, you can feel that way about exercise, too.

• *No energy.* This is the second-most common excuse. But the truth is that exercise will leave you feeling much more energized than watching *Mr. Ed* reruns.

• *No place to work out.* Exercising does not require membership in an expensive health club. Virtually every community has public facilities for sports and fitness. Be-sides, you can get a great workout in and around your home with weight lifting, calisthenics, running, walking and cycling.

• *No know-how.* Maybe you believe athletics are in-siderish, the exclusive realm of guys with an innate jock knowledge. Well, arm yourself with information. You picked up this book, so you're on your way. Also, swing by the library, watch for listings of exercise clinics, drop by a fitness fair and check out a video or the TV schedule for shows by credible fitness experts. Don't judge a video by the celebrity on the cover. Make sure the program has been developed or hosted by someone who is educated in the field and who is certified by organizations such as the National Strength and Conditioning Association or the American College of Sports Medicine.

go skiing occasionally. Exercise should be fun. Or at the least it has to be tolerable," says Dr. Chris Melby of the Human Energy Laboratory at Colorado State University. "Too many people start a program, they don't enjoy it and they quit. I just have learned to enjoy exercise, to find the things I really like to do, and so the motivation factor is there."

Here are some techniques for making your workout something to look forward to.

Make it different. A little variety will help hold your interest in working out. If your jogging's in a rut, find a new track or a path through the woods. Or try cross-training for a while: Take up cycling, swimming or karate.

If your weight lifting is getting tedious, change one of these factors.

- Frequency: how often you do an exercise, or the number of reps you do
- Intensity: the speed or the amount of weight you use
- Time: the duration of a particular exercise, or the number of sets you do

Involve friends and family. Bringing along a workout partner, or your personal cheering section, can be an enormous boost. People surveyed by the President's Council on Physical Fitness and Sports said spouses were the strongest positive influence on sticking with exercise. Friends will keep you in the game, too.

"The guys I play basketball with expect each other to be there," says Dr. Melby. "We enjoy the friendship as well as the exercise—something we can do together. There's a certain amount of accountability. If you don't show up, somebody from the group is going to get on the phone and say, 'Where are you?' "

Fight Discouragement

Tyranny is no fun. If once in a long while you blow off a workout in favor of an ice cream cone, accept it lightheartedly. Otherwise, the sense of failure can make it harder to get yourself back on track. Focus on how much

Spinning Cow Pies into Gold

Steve Urner's splendid throwing arm has always gotten him into deep doo-doo.

As a youngster growing up in Bakersfield, California, he earned a swat on the bottom for tossing a rock through the open window of a passing car. Tin can lids, he discovered, made dandy flying saucers. And when his sister got him mad, he'd fling a few of her Beatles 45s off the bluff near their house.

As a young man, he put his arm to slightly better use. The guys working a used-car lot near his job would take sucker bets from visitors and then summon the five-foot-ten-inch kid with the bionic arm to chuck a golf ball over an eight-story building.

At age 36 he flung himself into the record books. "I heard about this contest in the town of Tehachapi," recalls Urner, now a deputy sheriff and a real-estate broker. "Every year, they have a mountain festival, and they had a cow-chip throwing contest. I thought, 'You know, here's something I can do.' "

progress you've made so far, not on how far you have to go.

Here are additional ways to keep on keeping on.

Expect a slump. If you're feeling discouraged a few weeks into a new workout, don't give up—that's just a predictable part of the cycle, say fitness experts. You're no longer a novice in the gym, but you're surrounded by guys with rippling muscles while your flesh just kind of waggles. Your body's going through big changes—give it time.

Forget the scales. Don't try to chart your progress by weighing in. Sure you're losing fat, but you're also gaining muscle, which is heavier stuff. You could gain weight even though you're making advancements. If the

He selected a flat, dry beaut of a cow patty from the truckload at the festival—"just a real good one, one in a thousand." With a stiff wind at his back, he side-armed his prized bovine discus 266 feet and made his mark in the Guinness Book of World Records.

Oh, the celebrity! Parades, TV coverage, radio talk shows. A Japanese film crew even flew him to another festival in Beaver, Oklahoma, to fling some Sooner poop in a contest there.

In a bid for more credibility, Urner took a gold medal in the javelin in the California Police Olympics and went on to capture a silver medal in the nationals. "So my next feat, naturally, is to spear a cow chip *with* a javelin," he says.

Jokes aside, Urner is serious about goal-setting and achievement. "People who have their lives in order and have a regimen and a focus are going to have a better future," he says. "Positive mental attitude, being polite, working with people and asking their cooperation is all-important. Power to me is as simple as that."

'Whether you think you *can* or you think you *can't*, you're always right,'" says DeJesus.

Imagine the advantages of channeling this powerful mind-body connection to your favor. Studies show that athletes perform better when they banish negative thinking and immerse themselves in their objectives.

Psychologists at Springfield College in Springfield, Massachusetts, studied 24 junior tennis players during tournament play. Statistical analysis showed that players who berated themselves with cries like "Why can't I serve?" and "I'm so sloppy today!" followed up with even poorer performance. Bottom line: Practice mind over mutter.

Some athletes swear by meditation as a way of shouldering aside negativity and tapping inner power. "Meditation for me was the way that this all started—that's my motivation," says Furman, who has broken more than 40 Guinness records since he began studying the Eastern philosophy of teacher Sri Chinmoy.

If meditation is too mystic for your taste, there are alternatives. A mental exercise called visualization can rally both your mind and body toward reaching your goals. To do it, find a quiet place, breathe deeply and slowly, and relax thoroughly. Start by mentally counting down from 100, 50 or 25, seeing and hearing each number in your head.

Then mentally project yourself into the future. Imagine precisely how it will look and feel when you achieve your goal. If you want to bench-press a specific weight, picture the barbell above you, the feel of the bench against your back, the trickle of sweat on your brow.

Training experts say your subconscious mind will store such images and prime your body to physically re-create them when it's time for that big lift. Be patient with visualization—it takes practice.

scales are your only measure of progress, you might end up wrongly discouraged.

Schedule your workout. If you exercise on the same days at the same time, your routine will become a fixture in your life, not a whim. *Not* hitting the gym will feel unnatural.

Play Head Games

The mind just won't leave the body alone. Anxiety and negative thinking, for instance, can translate into physical problems like nausea and headaches. It also can cripple your performance as an athlete or render you so dispirited that you abandon your goals.

"I once heard a motivational coach say,

Power Tools

*Equipping Yourself
for Peak Performance*

Push-ups, crunches and calisthenics are all well and good, but if you truly want to start building strength, you're going to have to use more than your body. You're going to have to use your head.

That means learning about the equipment and accessories that will make you stronger. And they run the gamut, from simple tools with one function to massive contraptions so elaborate you'd think Rube Goldberg designed them. But believe it—every equipment or accessory choice you make, from the shoes on your feet to the weights you heft on your back, can have a direct impact on your fitness. Here's an overview of what you must have, as well as what you might want.

Hurry Up and Weight

Perhaps more than any other item, free weights will be the weapons of choice in your quest for power. And well they should be—nothing will make you powerfully fit faster.

"The fact is, you can get a more complete workout with free weights than machine weights. Machine weights are supported by the machine. Free weights are supported only by your muscles," says Steven McCaw, Ph.D., associate professor of biomechanics at Illinois State University in Normal. Dr. McCaw and his colleague Jeff Friday, a strength and conditioning coach at Northwestern University in

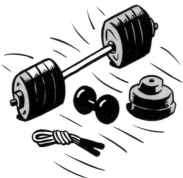

Evanston, Illinois, studied the differences between machine and free weights and found that exercisers actually used more muscles when they exercised with free weights. "There are a lot of secondary muscles that get exercised with free weights that you just don't use on a machine," Dr. McCaw says.

But all free weights are not necessarily created equal. There may be vast differences between the ones in the gym, the set on sale in the sporting goods store and the plastic, sand-filled barbell set you left in your parents' basement. Exercise experts and equipment designers weighed in with their insights—here's what they say to look for when it comes to pulling your own weights.

Be an Olympic lifter. In the world of free weights, experts agree the gold medal goes to the cast-iron Olympic weight set.

"It's a nice, basic design, very straightforward and easy to use. And if you're buying weights for a home gym, you can get a completely affordable package of weights that will let you do a lot of different exercises," says Tim Krivanek, an equipment designer for National Barbell Supply in Cleveland, Ohio. A basic Olympic set includes 255 pounds of weight plates, a 45-pound straight bar and two spring clips. Prices for the basic set range from $100 to $300, so shop around. "Then, you can always buy additional weight plates to augment your workout—they'll run you about 40 to 50 cents a pound," Krivanek says. That's cheaper than hamburger, and not nearly so fattening.

Clamp down. To keep those weight plates from sliding off the bar, make sure you use spring-loaded collars. "The screw-on clamps are a pain to remove—that makes it harder to change weights for different exercises," says Krivanek. With a spring-loaded collar, you just squeeze it, slip it on the bar and let go. Most basic weight sets come with two clamps—replacements can cost $10 to $20.

Be a benchwarmer. Don't even bother buying weights unless you're going to buy a bench.

"A free-weight barbell set isn't much good without a bench. You can't do a good workout unless you have one," says John Amberge, an exercise physiologist at the Sports Training Institute in New York City. Plus, there's a safety aspect to think about: If you're all alone in the basement and you suddenly need to set that barbell somewhere, where do you put it? That's why experts recommend an Olympic power bench, which has safety catches—vertical posts with several brackets to rack the weight off at various points if you're unable to complete the full range of motion. By itself, an Olympic bench with safety standards will set you back about $400 to $500, but equipment expert Krivanek says you can save money on a total weight-and-bench system if you negotiate a package deal.

"Some stores have a regular deal where, if you buy a bench, they'll give you the weights for, say, $99. If the place where you're shopping doesn't advertise a deal like that, ask the salesperson anyway—most stores will give you a break," he says.

Learn from dumbbells. Even after they've invested in the Olympic weight set and bench, smart lifters add a few dumbbells.

"What's nice about dumbbells is that they give you a little more range of motion than the basic weight set. When you're doing a flat bench press with a barbell, for example, you can only come down so far before the bar hits you in the chest," Krivanek says. "With dumbbells, you can go down just a little bit more, getting that greater range, that greater stretch." Plus, you can exercise each arm

individually, which keeps your dominant hand from doing most of the work. Start with four dumbbells: two 15-pounders and two 25-pounders. All four will run you about $50 total.

Completing the Circuit

Although free weights are the best line of defense against a flab onslaught, machine weights—circuit-training machines and home gym systems—do have their place in a workout.

"If you belong to a club and you have

When to Wear a Belt

According to Norse mythology, the thunder god Thor owned a magic belt. Whenever he strapped it on, he was endowed with fantastic strength, which came in pretty handy against trolls and frost giants.

Today, weight lifters like to think they have a magic belt that makes them stronger, too. It's called a weight belt—a big slab of leather you wrap around your lower back. For decades bodybuilders have sworn by them, but now some exercise experts are saying you should swear them off. Because just like Thor and his magic belt, the reputation of weight belts is based more on myth than fact.

"They may protect the back in certain exercises, if worn correctly," says Illinois State University's Dr. Steven McCaw. The problem is that many lifters end up using the belt as a crutch, relying on it to help them lift weights, when what they really should be doing is strengthening the muscles around the spine. About the only time to wear a weight belt is when you're doing bent-over lifts such as squat rows or any overhead lifts, such as military presses. Otherwise, keep that belt off your back.

access to circuit machines, or you already own a home gym, there's no reason not to incorporate it into your workout," Dr. McCaw says. While you work more muscles on free weights, machine weights allow you to work safely with heavier weights. The machine prevents the loaded bar from falling and crushing your body.

In the home gym arena there's a raft of styles, technologies and prices. Here's a thumbnail sketch of the different systems and an idea of what they'll cost you.

• *Weight-stack systems.* As close as you'll come to the machines at a health club, home gyms with weight stacks can give you the most professional workout. "Some are just as good as what you'll find in a fitness club, and, again, a machine weight system like that ensures a smooth, stable, safe lift," says Krivanek. But you get what you pay for—weight-stack systems start at around $700.

• *Body-weight systems.* The least expensive systems—running $300 to $500—often don't involve weights at all. "Some low-end ones rely on your body weight," says Krivanek. You sit on a bench, lift the bar and suddenly, the bench—and you—are moving up and down. You can change the resistance by adjusting the fulcrum that seesaws your body up and down. As body-weight exercises go, it's cheaper to do sit-ups and push-ups.

• *Other resistance systems.* Because weight stacks are so expensive and less costly body-weight systems may not give you enough of a workout, some manufacturers hit a happy medium with home gyms that rely on some type of resistance-applying device, such as flexible rods, rubber weight straps or hydraulic cylinders. The main difference among these systems, says Krivanek, is the feel of the motion. "The disadvantage to the resistance-type home gym is the lack of durability. Component parts will wear out faster," he says. On the other hand, these mid-range systems are convenient and relatively affordable—$500 to $1,000—and are fine if you're looking for a modest, maintenance workout.

Outfitting for Fitness

Clothes make the man, but they also can make the most of your workout. With the proper clothes you can keep your body temperature consistent, preventing overheating. Plus, the gear you choose for your hands and feet can help you keep a grip on the surfaces you're working out on.

"The more comfortable and appropriate the clothing, the better you'll feel when you're exercising," says Budd Coates, *Men's Health* magazine fitness consultant. And, as Coates points out, some apparel is absolutely essential for a safe workout. Here's a sample of your wardrobe options.

Break out in sweats. Heavy cotton sweatshirts, shorts and pants are perennial favorites. Nice and loose, they also soak up sweat, which keeps you from feeling too funky. Don't overwear sweat clothes in a feeble attempt to sweat off flab. "You'll just overheat yourself," Coates says.

Learn to like Lycra. The latest synthetic fabrics—nonabsorbent polyesters like Lycra—do a great job at wicking away moisture from your body. That's important—it helps to regulate your body temperature. The drawback: If you're not used to it, this high-tech clothing can seem constricting and slimy—or worse, make you feel like a refugee from a Richard Simmons video. No one's saying you have to wear butt-floss—just get a pair of Lycra shorts and wear a T-shirt or sweatshirt to cover them. No one's looking at you—trust us.

But if you just can't get used to the feel of Lycra, Coates recommends the tried-and-true cotton shorts and T-shirt wardrobe. "Cotton is really the best material for absorbing perspiration during workouts," says Coates, "and it's cooler."

Get a grip. When you're lifting weights, get yourself a pair of padded, fingerless, leather weight-lifting gloves (about $12 to $20 a pair). Besides saving your hands from countless blisters, they'll help you keep a tight grip on the bar. Also, they make you look like a fitness god.

Support cross-trainers. Obviously, depending on which sport you play, you'll need different foot gear—high-tops for hard-on-the-ankle sports like basketball, for example, or shoes with a balance of cushioning and support for running. But for your weighty workouts, you might want to look at a good pair of cross-trainers.

"Mid-cut cross-trainers provide a good base of support, which is important when you're lifting weights. Plus, you have cushioning for those dynamic activities in the weight room," says Tom Brunick, director of the Athlete's Foot Weartest Center at North Central College in Naperville, Illinois, and footwear editor for *Runner's World* magazine. "You can do a little bit of everything with a shoe like that. You can do weights, then jump on the stair-climbing machine, for example."

Go for Heavy Breathing

Manly as pumping iron may be, you're going to have to devote some time to getting your heart pumping. And if weather conditions or time constraints keep you indoors, that means exercising with devices that look like they're doing all the work for you—we're talking about aerobic machines and accessories here.

"These machines help to train your cardiovascular system, which is as important—if not more important—than just weight training," Amberge says. Weight training may get your heart beating faster and make your breathing heavier, but it doesn't get your heart rate up to the consistent, higher training level that's so important for keeping your cardiovascular system healthy.

Remember: Strong muscles are worthless

Step Up or Slide Over

Way over on the other side of the club, you may have noticed those Lycra-clad bodies hopping up and down or sliding side to side and wondered: What the heck are they doing?

It's called slide- and step-aerobics, and they're exercises that involve equipment you might want to add to your workout.

"Steps work like stair-climbing machines, only they're not as mechanical," says John Amberge of the Sports Training Institute. You step up and down at varying rhythms on the steps, which usually come in adjustable heights.

Slides, meanwhile, are rectangular plastic or vinyl strips you slide from side to side on, mimicking the motions of skating. "Slides are good because they enhance your balance skills and improve leg strength," Amberge says. "Both are great for improving heart and lung capacity and are great warm-up exercises before weight training."

---

if your heart and lungs aren't powerful enough to let you use them. Here's a quick rundown on the most common devices for an aerobic workout.

• *Treadmill.* Experts say this is one of the most popular machines, especially for men. This is no doubt because of the collective memory of watching the Six Million Dollar Man hit 60 miles per hour every week on *his* treadmill. Granted, you won't need the mile-a-minute setting on the average treadmill, but you can see how fast and how far you're running, which is nice. Plus, you can increase or decrease the pace or the incline of the treadmill belt so you can have an "uphill" workout. Best of all, some of these devices feature handy emergency shut-off switches so you won't end up like another TV icon, George Jetson, yelling for Jane to stop this crazy thing. A basic treadmill—nothing more than a conveyor belt with handles—costs a couple hundred bucks. You don't need to be the Six Million Dollar Man to afford higher-end models with inclines, digital readouts and built-in heart-rate monitors. But they are selling briskly above the $1,300 mark.

- *Stair-climber.* This one's easy to learn and doesn't require a ton of coordination. You can program it for different levels of difficulty, and some models even monitor calorie burn-off and heart rate. Prices range from about $1,000 to more than $2,000. You may find one significantly cheaper, but try it before you buy it. Many of the smaller steppers don't have a wide support base. The result is that they're unstable and have been known to flip over in the heat of a furious workout.

- *Stationary cycle.* Great for times when your schedule or the weather forbids a bike ride, newer cycling machines even have heart-rate monitors built in. Grip the handles and you'll get a reading. If you're not up for the expense—cycles with heart-rate monitors and other bells and whistles will run you around $1,000 or more—Amberge suggests checking your local bike or sporting goods shop for a wind trainer or a turbo-trainer. Many stores also sell a roller wheel that positions the rear wheel of your road bike off the floor, converting it into a stationary bike at home, for a little more than $100.

- *Rower.* A powerful workout machine not just for your heart and lungs, but also for your arms, legs and back. Our favorite models feature a built-in viewscreen that allows you to race against an onscreen opponent. Prices range from $200 for a basic model to well over $1,000 for the built-in arcade game.

- *Cross-country skier.* One of the most aerobic machines around, cross-country skiers can also be one of the most finicky. "They're great because they mimic the actions of cross-country skiing, which is tremendously aerobic," Amberge says. But the machines, like the sport, take some getting used to, since your feet are sliding backwards at the same time that your arms are swinging forward. Expect to spend around $600 to $800.

Exercise Extras

Some exercise equipment isn't vital to your fitness, but it sure makes life easier. And easy is good. After all, exercising with weights is hard, sweaty work. But having some convenient and helpful extras handy can make exercising almost fun. Here's a sampling of items you might be glad to have.

Hit the mat. Experts agree you shouldn't do any floor exercises on a hard, unyielding surface. Instead, use an exercise mat. Cheap—some cost about $10—convenient, easy on the body, an exercise mat is great for doing crunches, stretches and other calisthenics anytime and—since you can roll it up and stash it in a duffel bag—anywhere.

Give yourself enough rope. Another take-anywhere bit of equipment is a jump rope. It can improve your balance when you're weight training and give you explosive power in your favorite sports. As if that's not enough, jumping rope also makes a great exercise for your heart and lungs. But watch the surface you're jumping on, Dr. McCaw cautions. Look for soft flooring, not concrete.

Weigh in. Ankle and wrist weights ($10 to $15 a pair) can turn a minor exercise into a major muscle-builder. Doing moderate exercises with slow motion is the key. "Swing around too much while you're wearing weights—say while you're running or doing jumping jacks—and you can damage muscles and joints," warns Dr. McCaw. On the other hand, wearing weights while doing chin-ups can magnify your workout so you're lifting more than just body weight.

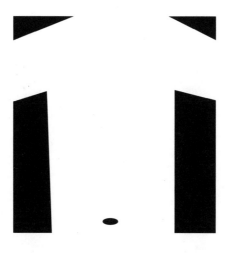

Part Two

Power Where
You Need It

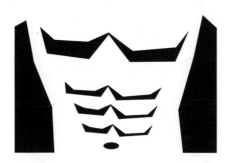

Abs

In the 1994 comedy *Junior*, viewers were treated to the spectacle of Arnold Schwarzenegger waddling around on-screen with a bulging belly. Thanks to the magic of movies, the former Mr. Universe was made pregnant.

That's a better excuse than most guys have for their potbellies. But it may provide some solace that, at least in his film role, Schwarzenegger got to experience what men with extra weight around their midsections are forced to live with—aching backs, sore legs and waddling walks.

Seventy-eight percent of American men are overweight, and that excess poundage piles up first around a guy's gut. That places a tremendous strain on the back.

"It's important to keep your lower back in mind if you carry excess weight around your midsection," says Richard T. Cotton, editor-in-chief for the American Council on Exercise's publication *ACE Fitness Matters*. "That added weight forces your lower back to arch, and this increases your risk for back pain and injury because it makes it harder for you to keep your back in a natural, neutral position."

A Six-Pack to Go

Your abs are actually several muscle groups, all located in the midsection from just below your chest to past your waistline.

The stomach muscle that gets the most attention is the *rectus abdominis*, the one responsible for the defined "six-pack" look that most guys crave. The rectus starts near the middle of your sternum and runs verti-

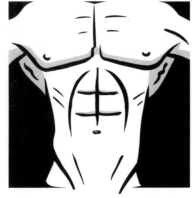

cally to the lower part of your pelvis. It's responsible for helping you curl your trunk, as you would while doing crunches.

The *transversus abdominis* is a deep muscle and the only abdominal muscle whose fibers run horizontally. It runs around your body much like a girdle and has a similar function too: It helps compress and support internal organs.

Then there are the obliques, but we'll give those special attention later.

Be an Abdominal Showman

We won't lie. Giving birth to a rock-hard stomach isn't easy. It takes effort and dedication. But it isn't impossible. And the benefits are twofold: Not only will your abs look like a bas-relief sculpture, the rest of your body—including your back—will feel better.

A word on the exercises. Abs are about the only muscles you can work every day, so don't feel you need to take it easy on them. Keep in mind that some experts have found that the upper ab muscles work 90 to 100 percent of their maximum ability in crunch exercises, but only about 30 percent in pelvic lift exercises. In contrast, pelvic lifts work the lower abs at about 80 percent, but the upper abs at only 30 percent. Knowing this will help you target which exercises to use for each muscle.

And finally, a word on hand positioning for crunches. Despite what your gym teacher told you, don't lock your hands behind your head. Yanking your head up may hurt your neck or back. Instead, cup your fingertips behind your ears. Or, if you find that too difficult, try folding your hands across your chest.

Here are some great exercises to help you work your way into middle management.

Upper and Lower Abs
Curl-Ups

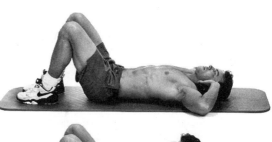

Lie flat on your back with your fingertips cupped behind your ears. Keep your feet together, flat on the floor and about six inches from your butt. Bend your knees at about a 45-degree angle, and keep your legs slightly apart.

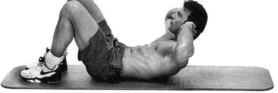

Without moving your lower body, curl your upper torso up and in toward your knees until your shoulder blades are as high off the ground as you can get them. Only your shoulders should lift—not your back. Feel your abs contract, and hold the raise for a second. Lower to the starting position, then continue with your next rep without relaxing in between.

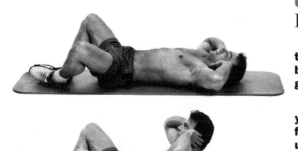

Upper and Lower Abs
Frog-Leg Crunches

Lie flat on your back with knees spread and the soles of your feet together. Your knees should be as close to the floor as you comfortably can get them. Cup your fingertips behind your ears.

Keeping the rest of your body in place, lift your shoulder blades and upper back off the floor. At the same time slightly curl your pelvis up and in, but don't lift your lower back off the floor. Concentrate on your ab contraction. Hold for a second, then lower to the starting position. Don't rest when you're done. Repeat your next rep, keeping your abs tight.

Upper and Lower Abs, Obliques
Crossover Crunches

Lie flat on your back in crunch position, with your feet flat and your knees up. Keep your feet about hip-width apart and cup your fingertips behind your ears.

Raise your trunk up, lifting your shoulders and shoulder blades off the ground. But instead of pausing at the top, slightly twist toward your left knee. Hold the contraction for a split second, then lower to the starting position. Repeat, but this time twist to your right knee. Don't relax between reps.

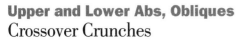
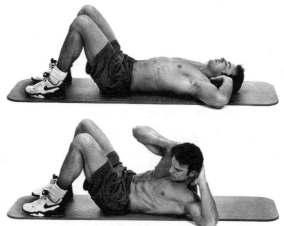

Note: The difference between crunches and curl-ups, according to physical therapist and fitness consultant Deborah Ellison of San Diego, California, is that crunches involve a pelvic tilt, so your body is almost folding in on itself at the midsection. Curl-ups are a bit easier because the top part of your body is simply curling in toward your midsection. There's no pelvic action.

Upper and Lower Abs
Raised-Leg Crunches

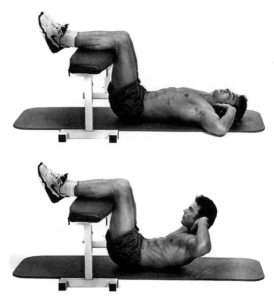

Lie on your back with your knees bent and your legs up on a bench or chair. Your thighs should be perpendicular to the floor, and your fingertips cupped behind your ears.

Lift your torso up and in toward your knees, lifting your shoulders and shoulder blades off the floor. Hold the contraction for a second, then lower to the starting position. Repeat, but don't relax between reps.

Variation: Can also be done without a chair if you have enough muscle strength to hold your legs up in the air without support.

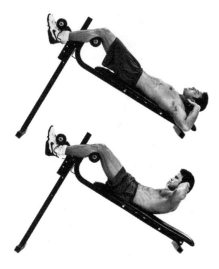

Upper and Lower Abs
Decline Crunches

Lie on your back on a decline board, with your ankles hooked under the padded support bars and your fingertips cupped behind your ears. The decline board provides more resistance since you're fighting gravity on the way up.

Raise your shoulder blades up off the bench, keeping your lower back flat. Don't jerk your body to build momentum. Hold the contraction for a second, then lower to the starting position. Repeat, but don't relax between reps.

Upper and Lower Abs
Hanging Single-Knee Raises

Hang fully extended from a chin-up bar with your palms facing out and your hands a little wider than shoulder-width apart. Your feet should be lightly touching the floor.

Without swinging to pick up momentum, raise your right knee toward your left shoulder as far as you can, using your abs for power. Slightly thrust your pelvis forward to help, but don't rock. Hold for a second, then lower to the starting position and repeat with your left leg. Don't relax between sets.

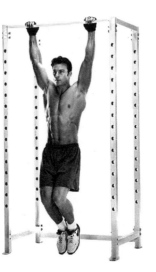
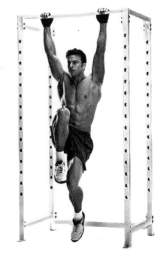

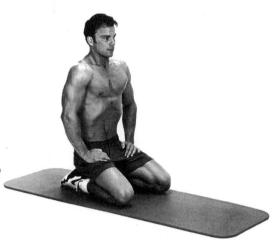

Upper and Lower Abs
Vacuums

Sit in a kneeling position with your hands on your thighs. Keep your upper body upright. Breathe out, then immediately suck your stomach up and in as far as it will go. Hold for ten seconds. Repeat.

***Note:* You can increase the "vacuum" time to up to 30 seconds as your stomach gets stronger. You can also do this exercise from a standing position.**

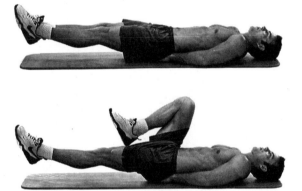

Upper and Lower Abs
Raised-Leg Knee-Ins

Lie on your back on the floor. Your arms should be close to your sides, with your hands palm-down and just under your lower back and butt. Press the small of your back against the floor and extend your legs outward with your heels about three inches above the floor.

Keeping your lower back against the floor, lift your right knee toward your chest, keeping your left leg hovering above the floor. Hold, then straighten your leg to the starting position and repeat with the other leg. Keep your abs taut throughout the exercise.

Upper and Lower Abs
V-spread Toe Touches

Lie flat on your back with your legs straight up in a V-position; don't lock your knees. Raise your arms to the ceiling.

Curl your shoulder blades up and reach toward your left foot. Hold for a second, concentrating on your abs, then lower to the starting position. Repeat, this time reaching for the right foot. Don't pause at the lower position. Keep your abs tight.

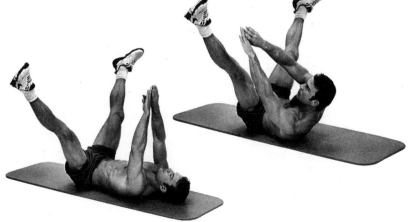

The Underappreciated Obliques

Your obliques are the stomach muscles that make up your waist. The external oblique (*obliquus externus abdominis*) is the muscle of the upper and outside part of your waistline. It starts just under your chest, on your lower eight ribs, and is responsible for helping you twist and bend sideways. The right external oblique helps you twist left, and vice versa. The internal oblique (*obliquus internus abdominis*) is similar, but it's situated underneath the external oblique. It, too, helps you twist and bend. The right internal oblique helps you twist to the right, and vice versa.

In most men these fine strips of beef are often covered with fat. That's a shame, says physical therapist Deborah Ellison.

"The stomach muscles that I feel are most important are the obliques," says Ellison, a former kinesiology teacher at San Diego State University and a current health writer and adviser to the American Council on Exercise. "Yet most people spend their time working the rectus for that cut-up washboard look. That looks good, but it doesn't do as much for your back or for helping control intra-abdominal pressure."

Here are two excellent ways to give your obliques the attention they deserve.

Obliques
Oblique Twists

Stand upright with your feet about shoulder-width apart and your knees unlocked. Hold a broomstick across your shoulders, behind your neck so it's resting on your trapezius and upper deltoid muscles. Your hands should be grasping the ends of the broomstick, or as close to the ends as you can get them.

Keeping your hips still and facing forward, twist to your left as far as you can go. Then twist in the opposite direction. Keep a slow, steady pace and concentrate on working your obliques.

Obliques
Oblique Crunches

Lie flat on your back with your knees bent and your fingertips cupped behind your ears. Now let your legs fall as far as they can to your right side, so that your upper body is now flat on the floor and your lower body is on its side.

Keeping your shoulders as close to parallel to the floor as possible, lift your upper body up until your shoulder blades clear the ground. Concentrate on the oblique contraction and hold the crunch for a second. Then lower to the starting position and do your next rep. Don't rest between crunches—keep your abs tight. After one set on your right side, switch to your left and continue.

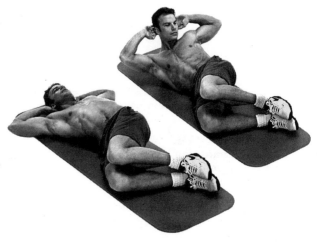

The ⬆ next level

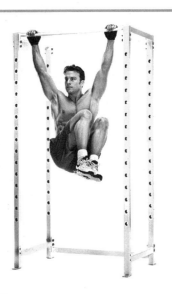

Upper and Lower Abs, Obliques:
Hanging Knee Raise Crossovers

Hang fully extended from a chin-up bar with your hands a little wider than shoulder-width apart. Your palms should be facing outward and your feet lightly touching the floor. Now, keeping your legs together, slowly lift your knees up toward your left shoulder as high as you can. Slightly thrust your pelvis forward, but don't rock or sway for momentum. Hold for a second at the top, then lower and repeat on your right side. Don't rest between reps. Keep your abs tight.

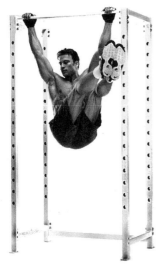

Upper and Lower Abs, Obliques:
Hanging Leg Raise Crossovers

Hang fully extended from a chin-up bar with your hands a little wider than shoulder-width apart. Your palms should be facing outward and your feet lightly touching the floor. Now slowly lift your legs, feet together, toward your left shoulder as high as you can so your legs are roughly at a 45-degree angle. You'll need to slightly tilt your pelvis forward. Lower, then repeat on the right side. Don't rest between reps. Keep your abs tight.

Obliques: Dumbbell Sidebends

Stand upright with a dumbbell in each hand. Your feet should be about shoulder-width apart, and your arms should be resting at your sides with your palms facing in.

Bend to one side, allowing the dumbbell to drop down your leg until you feel your obliques working. Keep your body facing front in the same plane—don't turn your torso into the sidebend. Once you've gone as low as you can, slowly bring yourself upright to the starting position and repeat. Don't rest between reps. Keep your abs and obliques contracted. When you're done with one side, work the other.

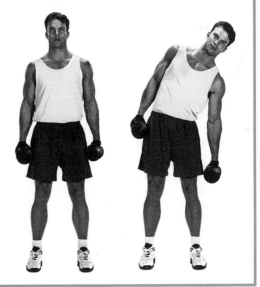

Legs

You don't need to be a soccer player or ballet dancer to appreciate your legs. Without them you couldn't climb stairs, sprint for meetings or bounce children on your knee. But in the gym, legs are like Rodney Dangerfield: They get no respect.

"Most guys don't work their legs as much as they should, and if they do, it's usually only on the extension machines so they can see their quads bulging," says Ed Burke, Ph.D., associate professor at the University of Colorado at Colorado Springs and vice-president of the National Strength and Conditioning Association.

Your legs, made up of four bones each, account for roughly 14 percent of your total body weight. At their core, each leg features the body's largest bone, the femur, which averages 19 inches in a six-foot man and comprises roughly 28 percent of his height.

Your legs also play host to the foot-long thigh muscles,

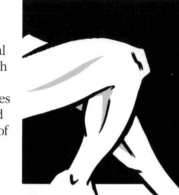

some of the largest muscles in your body. The muscles on the front of your thigh are called the quadriceps. They're so named because they're a grouping of four different muscles: the *rectus femoris, vastus lateralis, vastus medialis* and *vastus intermedialis.* The rectus femoris runs along the front of your thigh, crossing both your hip and knee joints. It flexes your hip and, along with the vastus muscles, extends your knee.

Bringing up the rear of your legs are the hamstring muscles. You probably first heard of these muscles in junior high football or track, since they're so often pulled or torn by athletes young and old alike. The hamstrings are a group of three muscles: the *biceps femoris,* the *semimembranosus* and *semitendinosus.* They run along the back of your legs, from your knee to your hips, where they cross the hip joint. Farther down on your legs, behind your shins, are the calf muscles, the *gastrocnemius* and *soleus,* both of which help flex your foot downward, which helps you walk, jump or sprint.

Here's how to get started making a stand for fitness.

Quadriceps
Leg Extensions

Sit in a leg extension machine, with your legs behind the padded lifting bars and your hands grasping the machine's handles or the sides of the bench. Your knees should be bent at 90 degrees or slightly more, with your toes pointing in front of you.

Using the machine's handles or the side of the bench for support, straighten your legs by lifting with your ankles and contracting your quads. Don't lock your knees at full extension, but rather keep a slight bend. Your toes should be pointing up and out at about a 45-degree angle.

***Variations:* Foot positioning changes the way your muscles are worked. Try pointing your toes back or straight to work different parts of your quads.**

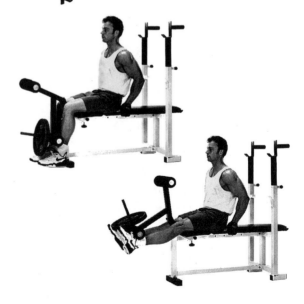

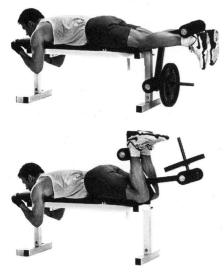

Hamstrings
Leg Curls

Lie on your stomach on a leg curl machine, with your ankles hooked behind the lifting pads and your knees just over the bench's edge. Hold onto the machine's handlebars, if any, for support. Your legs should be fully extended with some natural flex at the knee, and your toes should be pointing down.

Keeping your pelvis flush against the bench, raise your heels up toward your butt so that your legs bend to about a 90-degree angle. Use the handlebars for support, and keep your feet pointing away from your body.

***Note:* Some leg curl machines are bent slightly at the end to relieve pressure from your pelvis. If yours is not, consider placing a small pillow under your pelvis. Also, your hamstrings are weaker than your quads. Use less weight for leg curls than you would for leg extensions.**

Calf Muscles
Heel Raises

Stand with a dumbbell in each hand. Your feet should be hip-width apart with your toes on a platform raised a couple of inches off the ground. Your heels should be on the floor, and your weight should be on the balls of your feet so you're leaning forward slightly. Hold the dumbbells at your sides, with your arms extended down.

Rise all the way up onto your toes. Feel the contraction in your calves and pause briefly at the top. Your arms should remain in position, though your body will probably be more upright.

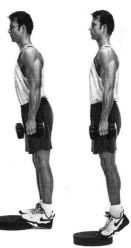

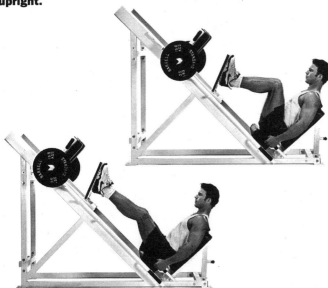

Quadriceps
Leg Presses

Sit in a leg press machine with your feet on the pedals in front of you. The seat should be adjusted so your knees are bent at about a 90-degree angle or a little straighter. Grasp the handlebars at your sides and hold your upper body upright, but relaxed.

Push forward on the foot plates and straighten your legs until they're fully extended in front of you. Keep your knees slightly flexed. Your upper body should remain upright and relaxed, and your hands should hold the handlebars for support.

Quadriceps
Dumbbell Lunges

Stand upright with a dumbbell in each hand. Your arms should be fully extended at your sides, your palms facing in. Your feet should be about hip-width apart, and your torso upright with your lower back maintaining a natural inward curve.

Step forward with your right leg slightly farther than you would in a normal step. Your upper body should remain upright and slightly forward, with your arms at your sides and the dumbbells roughly in the centerline of your body. Your lead leg should be bent at a 90-degree angle, so you can still see your toes if you look down at them. Your back leg should be slightly bent at the knee, but otherwise straight. The heel of your trailing foot will rise slightly, but your foot should remain in the same position. Return to original position.

***Note:* You can alternate lunges or do all on one leg, then switch legs. Try these also without weights or with a barbell.**

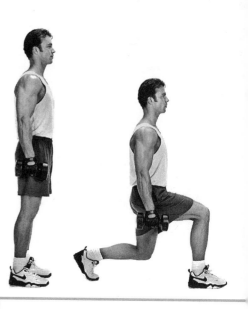

The ⬆ next level

Hip Flexors and Quadriceps:
Traditional Squats

Stand before a squat rack, grasping a barbell palms-down. Place it behind your neck and evenly across your trapezius and deltoids. Your torso should be erect, your feet hip-width apart with your toes forward and slightly out. Knees are slightly bent, and your lower back should have a slight forward lean.

Squat down as if sitting in a chair. Keep your shins close to perpendicular to the floor, and keep your balance centered and feet flat. Your thighs shouldn't exceed the point of being parallel to the floor. Your gaze should be forward, your upper torso slightly leaned forward and your lower back slightly curved inward or straight. Keep your feet flat on the floor and the barbell centered. Rise to the starting position.

Hip Flexors and Quadriceps:
Front Squats

Use the same technique as in a traditional squat, but grasp the bar with a palms-up grip, placing your hands equidistant from the center, shoulder-width apart. Elbows are pointing forward as the barbell rests across your upper chest and deltoids.

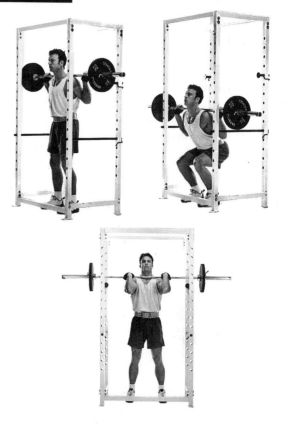

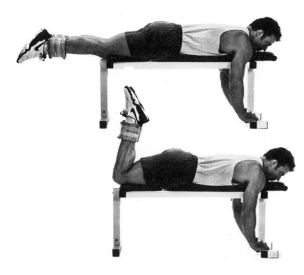

Hamstrings
Leg Curls with Cuff Weights

Lie on your stomach on a bench with both legs straight out and a cuff weight on each ankle. Your knees should be just past the bench's edge so you can bend your legs up. Your hands can be holding on to the bench's legs for support.

Keeping your feet together and pointed out, curl the weights in a semicircular motion toward your butt until your legs are at about a 90-degree angle. Point your toes up, and don't arch your pelvis or back. Your body should remain flush with the bench.

Quadriceps: **Barbell Step-Ups**

Hold a barbell behind your neck. Your palms should be facing out and the barbell should be even across your shoulders. Stand upright, with shoulders back, chest out and a slight forward lean in your lower back. Face a box that's 12 to 18 inches high; stand about a foot away. Make sure it's on a nonslip surface. The box should be high enough so your knee bends at about a 90-degree angle when you step on it.

Place your left foot in the center of the box. Your body should be erect, and the barbell should remain in position behind your neck.

Your weight should be shifted to your lead leg as your trailing foot steps up, bringing you to a standing position on top of the box with your feet together in the center.

Step backward so the foot of your trailing leg is near the starting position, then step down with the lead foot. Repeat with your other leg.

Note: This also can be done with dumbbells.

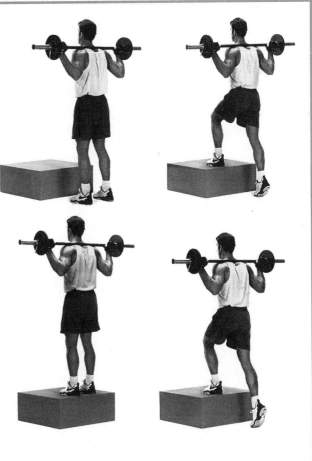

Butt

For some guys the main function of the butt is to leave a permanent indentation on the sofa. But in the hustle and bustle of daily life, the butt's a key player in nearly everything you do, whether you're pedaling cross-country on a bike or just sitting down at the end of a long day. You might call the butt your seat of power.

"In cycling, for example, the power muscles are the butt muscles. They're the biggest group of muscles used and probably the most important," says Dr. Ed Burke of the University of Colorado.

Power to the Max

Your butt muscles come in three sizes: the *gluteus maximus*, *gluteus medius* and the *gluteus minimus*. These glutes are made for walking—and

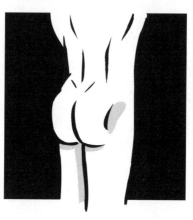

more. The maximus, as you can guess by its name, is the biggest and most noticeable of the three. The medius and the minimus aren't as eye-catching. Both are located around your ilium, the large bony upper part of your pelvis. Together, these three musketeers of muscle help move your thigh out to the side of your body, as well as rotate and extend your legs behind you.

Although no one wants a weather balloon for a butt, size isn't really the issue. You should be more concerned with how toned it is. A strong butt helps build explosive power in your lower body, Dr. Burke says. Plus, there's an added benefit. Research shows strong glutes can alleviate back pain. So if you're among the 80 percent of American men who suffer from an aching lower back, working these muscles will take you off the disabled list. No ifs, ands or butts about it.

Here's how to maximize your maximus and build glute strength.

Glutes
Pelvic Lifts

Lie on your back, with your knees bent and feet slightly apart, flat on the floor. Your arms should be at your sides, with your hands palms-down on the floor.

Lift your pelvis up toward the ceiling. Squeeze your butt together as you lift until your back is straight. Don't arch your back. Lower.

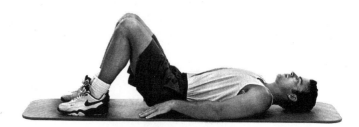

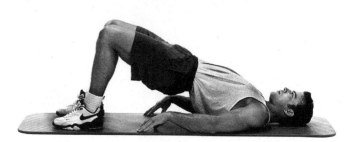

Glutes
Bent-Kick Crosses

Get down on the floor on all fours. Raise one leg several inches off the floor and bend it at roughly a 90-degree angle.

Push your leg up and back, reaching your heel to the ceiling. You should feel your butt contract as you push up. Your thigh should not go beyond being parallel with the floor and your leg should remain bent at a 90-degree angle. Lower. Finish your reps, then switch to the other leg.

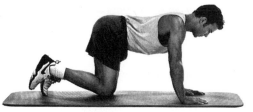

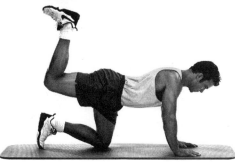

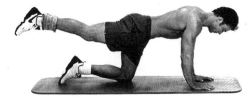

Glutes
Raised-Leg Curls

Get down on all fours on the floor wearing an ankle weight on your right leg. Raise your right leg to about butt level and extend it straight, away from your body and roughly parallel to the floor.

Curl your heel toward your butt, keeping your thigh level and parallel to the ground. Your thigh shouldn't move much—all the movement is done below the knee. Don't sway your body or arch your back, and concentrate on the contraction in your butt. When finished, switch the ankle weight to your left leg and repeat with that leg.

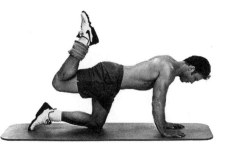

Glutes
Standing Kickbacks

Stand facing a wall, lightly holding on with your hands for balance. You should be wearing an ankle weight on one leg and leaning slightly forward so your whole body is in a straight line. Your weight should be shifted on the unweighted leg.

Move the weighted leg back as far as you can, feeling the contraction in your butt. Your knee should be slightly bent. Don't arch your back or overextend yourself. Hold, lower, repeat. When finished, place the ankle weight on the other leg and repeat.

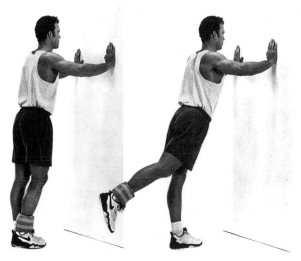

Chest

A sculpted chest is like an expensive tie or shined shoes: It does wonders for your image. "If you have a large chest, it helps to de-emphasize an overly fed stomach," says Thomas R. Baechle, Ed.D., professor of exercise science at Creighton University in Omaha, Nebraska, and executive director of certification for the National Strength and Conditioning Association.

Indeed, Canadian researchers who asked college-age men what caused them the most angst about their appearance found that puny pecs ranked right up top with waist size.

Your pecs are more than just showpieces. They're important functionally, too. Without pecs your arms would be far less useful, since your chest muscles help move them toward and away from your body. They also help flex and rotate your arms.

Unearthing a Treasured Chest

The chest muscles are an impressive lot. Endomorphs—people genetically predisposed to fleshiness—generally have the largest. T. J. Albert Jackson of Canton, Mississippi, has a chest that measures 120 inches.

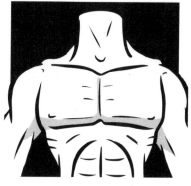

Of course, he weighs more than 800 pounds. The largest muscular chest belongs to Isaac Nesser of Greensburg, Pennsylvania. His pecs measure 74⅟₁₆ inches.

The chest muscles are called the pectorals, or pecs for short. The *pectoralis major* is the biggie. This thick, fan-shaped muscle spans most of your clavicle and sternum and attaches to your upper arm. There's also the *pectoralis minor*, a thin triangular muscle located beneath its big brother. The pecs differ from most other muscles because they're made of microscopic fibers that vary in length. Most muscles have fibers equal in length.

Before you try to move up in the pec-ing order, exercise caution in the weight room, advises James E. Graves, Ph.D., associate professor and chair of the Department of Health and Education at Syracuse University in New York. "Men in general are able to lift considerably more weight with their chest than they can in other upper-body exercises," he says. "The bench press is one of the typical exercises men like to show off with.

"Be careful when you're pushing heavy weight," Dr. Graves adds. "Chest exercises can be dangerous if you're trying to get maximal output without a partner or spotter."

Here's how to pump up your pec power.

Lower and Outer Pecs
Dips

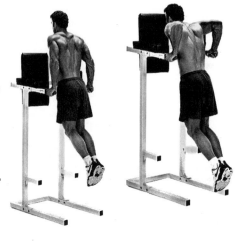

Raise yourself off the ground and onto parallel dip bars. Your hands should be gripping the bar handles with your fingers on the outside, facing away from your body. Keep your elbows in close to your sides, and slightly bend your legs if your feet are dragging on the ground.

Lower yourself down to the point where your upper arms are parallel to the floor. Keep your elbows close to your sides, and bend your legs slightly if your feet are touching the ground. Raise to the starting position.

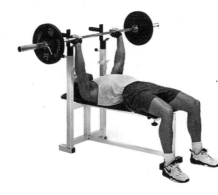

Middle Pecs
Bench Presses

Lie on a bench-press bench with the barbell above your chest. Grasp the barbell with a medium grip (hands about shoulder-width apart) or slightly wider. Your palms should face your legs, and your feet should rest on the ground. Keep your back straight and against the bench.

Lower the barbell to your nipple line. Your elbows should be pointed out while the rest of your body remains in position. Don't arch your back or bounce the bar off your chest. Raise to the starting position.

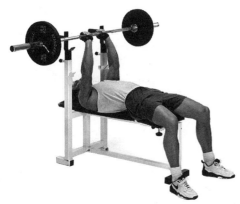

Lower and Inner Pecs
Narrow-Grip Bench Presses

Do a normal bench press with the proper form, but hold the barbell with a narrow grip. Your hands should be equidistant from the bar center, six to eight inches apart.

Note: Decrease the weight for this exercise, since it will be stressing your pecs from a different angle and you'll likely find it harder than standard presses.

Upper and Outer Pecs
Wide-Grip Bench Presses

Do a normal bench press with the proper form, but hold the barbell with a wide grip. Your hands should be equidistant from the bar center, a few inches wider than shoulder-width apart.

Note: Decrease the weight for this exercise, since it will be stressing your pecs from a different angle and you'll likely find it harder than standard presses.

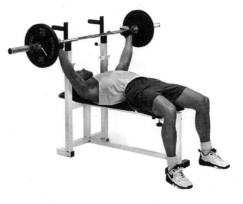

Upper and Outer Pecs
Inclined Bench Presses

Lie on an inclined bench-press bench with the barbell above your chest. Grasp the barbell with a medium grip (hands about shoulder-width apart) or slightly wider. Your palms should face your legs, and your feet should be on the ground. Keep your back against the bench.

Lower the barbell to your chest, between your shoulders and nipple line. Elbows should be pointing out, and the rest of your body should stay in proper form. Don't arch your back or bounce the bar off your chest.

Note: Wear a weight belt to give your back more support during this exercise.

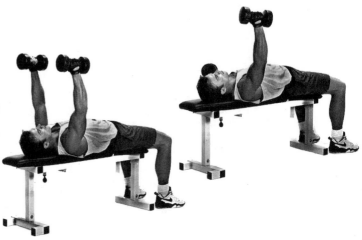

Outer and Upper Pecs
Dumbbell Flies

Lie on your back on a bench with your legs parted and feet firmly on the floor. Hold two dumbbells above you, palms facing each other. The dumbbells should be nearly touching each other above your chest. Your back should be straight and firm against the bench, and your elbows unlocked.

Slowly lower the dumbbells out and away from each other in a semi-circular motion. Keep your wrists locked. Lower until the dumbbells are at chest level. Your elbows should be bent at roughly a 45-degree angle, while your back is straight. Raise to the starting position.

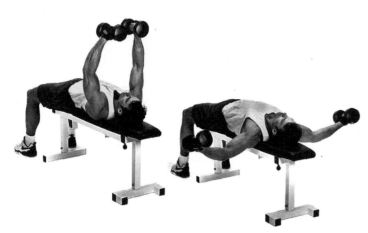

Middle Pecs
Alternating Dumbbell Presses

Grasp two dumbbells and lie back on a bench with your legs slightly parted, feet firmly on the floor and your arms raised. Hold the dumbbells above you, palms facing each other. The dumbbells should be about shoulder-width apart. Arms are extended, back is straight and firm against the bench and elbows are un-locked.

Lower the left dumbbell until it's even with your chest. Your elbow should be pointing to the ground. Raise to the starting position, then alternate with the right dumbbell.

Middle Pecs
Decline Push-Ups

Get in push-up position, but prop your feet up on a bench. Hands are roughly shoulder-width apart, and your back is straight. Keep your elbows unlocked.

Lower yourself to the floor as far as you can, or until your nose touches the ground. Your back and hips are straight, while your elbows point out. Keep your feet on the bench. Return to the starting position.

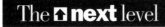

The ⌂ next level

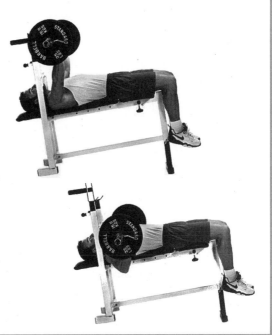

Middle Pecs: Push-Ups with Weights

Do a push-up with proper form, but have a partner place a weight plate squarely on your back for added resistance. The plate should be between your shoulder blades on your upper back.

Lower and Outer Pecs: Decline Bench Presses

Lie on a decline bench press with a barbell held above your body in preparation for the press. Grasp the barbell with a medium grip (hands about shoulder-width apart) or slightly wider. Your palms should be facing your legs, and your feet should be hooked under the support bar, if there is one. Keep your back straight and against the bench.

Lower the barbell to your nipple line, keeping your elbows pointed out. The rest of your body stays in proper starting form. Don't arch your back or bounce the bar off your chest. Raise to the starting position.

Note: Decline presses stress your chest from a different angle than standard presses, so decrease the weight.

Arms

Think back to when you were a kid. Back when Halloween was the only day of the year you used shaving cream. Chances are that sometime another kid asked—or dared—you to "make a muscle." What'd you do?

You raised your arm, bent your elbow and struck that archetypal bodybuilding pose you had seen countless times in ads in the back of comic books. And even though your prepubescent biceps barely bulged, the message was clear: Men should be well-armed.

You're not a kid anymore, but the message remains the same: When it comes to having a good body, well-defined arms are high on the list of Muscles That Matter.

Negotiating Your Own Arms Agreement

No doubt about it, the superstar muscles of your arms are the biceps and triceps. Although most guys probably never give it much thought, the names are anatomically descriptive: Biceps literally means "two heads." The biceps brachii is actually one muscle that branches into a long and a short head.

What people commonly refer to as the biceps actually are two distinct muscles: the *biceps brachii* and the *brachialis*. The biceps brachii is the one responsible for the "head" of your biceps. The brachialis is the larger of the two, and it's located underneath the biceps brachii. Both muscles help you flex your elbow, though the biceps brachii also comes into play when you move your shoulder.

When you talk about your triceps, you're actually referring to one muscle that has three "heads": the *caput longum,*

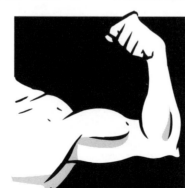

caput laterale and the *caput mediale.* It runs along the back side of your upper arm, opposite your biceps, and is responsible for extending your arm after it has been bent at the elbow.

Arming Yourself for Action

Exercising your right to bare arms can be extremely rewarding because you'll see noticeable results within a few weeks. Unfortunately, you'll also be tempted to speed up the process by working with too much weight too quickly. Well, don't. It'll only lead to poor technique, and poor technique robs your arms of a better workout. Plus it puts you at risk for pulling a muscle. So don't pile on the plates.

"It's better to grab something that's too light than to try to pick 100 pounds right off the bat," says John Skowron, a physical therapist at Raleigh Community Sports Medicine and Physical Therapy in Raleigh, North Carolina. "You can always go up in weight later. It's easier and safer to do that than to start out with too much."

And before you jump entirely on the biceps bandwagon, don't neglect those tri's. "Almost two-thirds of your arm is triceps, so if you really want nice-looking arms, don't forget there's a lot of meat there on the back of your arms," says Creighton University's Dr. Thomas R. Baechle. "Working triceps can really help increase the size of your arms."

Finally, this parting advice: Strong arms are enticing, but don't spend *all* of your workout time on them. "Sure they're nice to look at, but I think arms are sometimes given a bit too much attention," says Richard T. Cotton of the American Council on Exercise's publication *ACE Fitness Matters.* "There are a variety of other exercises that will do more for your body than just give you certain muscles to show off."

Here are some great exercises to build powerful arms.

Biceps
Barbell Curls

In a standing position grip the barbell with an underhand grip (palms facing up) with your hands about shoulder-width apart. Your arms should be extended and the barbell should be around your thighs. Your knees should be unlocked.

Keeping your elbows close to your body, use your biceps to curl the bar slowly up toward your chin. Keep your wrists straight throughout the curl, and don't sway your back or rock your body for momentum. Lower to the starting position.

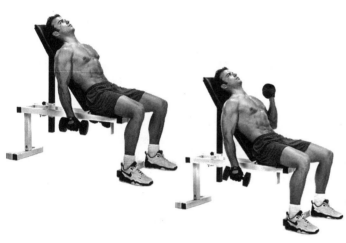

Biceps
Alternating Incline Dumbbell Curls

Lie on an incline bench with a dumbbell in each hand and your arms down at your sides. Hold the dumbbells in an overhand grip, with your palms facing in toward your body.

Curl the left-hand dumbbell up toward your biceps, keeping your wrist straight and being careful not to sway your shoulder to gain momentum. As you curl, slowly twist your wrist out so your palm is facing up toward the ceiling at the apex of the curl. Lower to the starting position and repeat with the right arm.

Biceps
Alternating Hammer Curls

Sit at the end of a bench with your feet slightly apart. You should be holding a dumbbell in each hand, with your palms facing your body. Your shoulders should be back and your upper torso upright.

Now curl the left dumbbell up in a semicircular motion toward your left biceps. You should not rock or sway to build momentum. Your wrist should be locked and your palm should continue to face in toward your body as you lift. Lower, then repeat with your right arm.

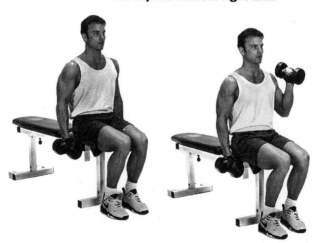

Biceps
Concentration Curls

Straddle the end of a bench holding a dumbbell in one hand. Your feet should be wider than shoulder-width apart and your knees bent. Bend forward and extend the arm holding the dumbbell between your legs so that your elbow and upper arm are braced against the inside of your thigh. The dumbbell should be held with a palm-up grip, and you should be leaning slightly into that side. Rest your other hand on your other knee.

Curl the dumbbell up toward your shoulder, bracing your elbow against your thigh and leaning on your other hand for support. Hold the curl, then lower with control. Finish your reps, then switch hands.

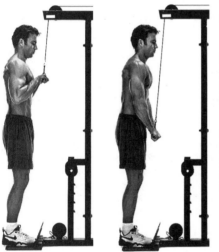

Triceps
Triceps Pull-Downs

Stand facing the triceps pull-down machine, gripping the handle with both hands, palms facing away from you in a narrow grip. Your hands should be gripping the bar as high as you can comfortably do it. Keep your elbows in by your sides and your upper arms perpendicular to the floor.

In a smooth motion pull down on the bar until you've straightened out both arms and they're pointing toward the floor. Your elbows should remain in close to your body, and you should feel the contraction in your triceps. Your wrists should be locked and straight. Raise the bar with control, returning to the starting position.

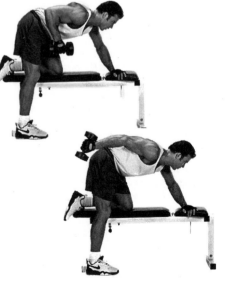

Triceps
Dumbbell Kickbacks

Start with a dumbbell in your right hand, with your palm facing in toward your body. Your right foot should be on the ground, your left knee and your left hand should rest on a bench for support. Bring the dumbbell up and into your body close to your left chest muscles. Your arm should be in close to your rib cage, with your elbow pointing up toward the ceiling. Your back should be straight and roughly parallel to the floor.

Resting on your left knee and hand, extend the dumbbell out and away from your body with your right arm. You should feel the contraction in your triceps. Extend your arm until it's straight and your triceps are fully contracted. Don't lean or sway or arch your back.

Triceps
Overhead Triceps Extensions

Lie on your back on a bench, holding a barbell above your chest with a narrow overhand grip (hands four to six inches apart) with palms facing up. Your feet should be up on the bench with feet together and legs slightly parted.

Bend your elbows, lowering the weight in a semicircle toward the top of your head. Raise to the starting position. Don't sway your arms through the motion. Concentrate on using only your triceps.

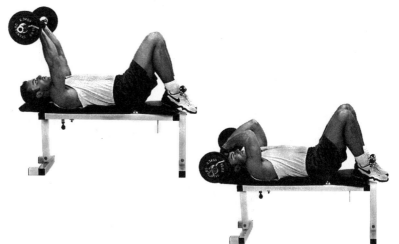

The ⌂ next level

Biceps: **Preacher Curls**

Sit in a preacher bench and hold a curling bar in both hands, with your arms over the bench platform. Your hands should be palms up, holding the bar about shoulder-width apart in a medium grip. Your feet should be firmly on the ground, your upper body upright and your eyes forward.

Raise the barbell in a semicircular motion toward your chin. Your elbows should stay put, and your wrists should be locked. Because your biceps are doing all the work, they get a more thorough (and tougher) workout.

Note: Lower your normal curling weight at first, since these curls are extra hard. You also can try them with dumbbells.

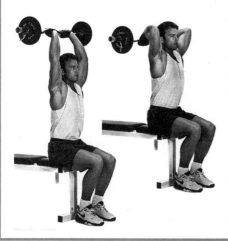

Triceps: **Seated Overhead Triceps Extensions**

Sit at the end of a bench with your feet firmly on the ground and a barbell held overhead with a narrow grip, palms facing out. Your upper torso should be erect and facing forward, with a slight natural forward lean in your lower back.

Keeping your upper body in place, lower the barbell behind your head. Keep your upper arms close to your head, and lower the bar in a semicircular motion until your forearms are as close to your biceps as possible. You might lean slightly forward to help offset the weight, but don't sway or arch your back. Your elbows should be facing forward. Raise to the starting position.

Back

Think of your back as Salvador Dali thought of a ten-foot canvas: It's a medium. But in this case, it's a medium of muscle just waiting to be turned into anatomical art.

"The back is beautiful. You have large muscles there working together with small muscles," says Jim Wichmann, an exercise physiologist and manager of an industrial rehabilitation program at Professional Sports Care in Paramus, New Jersey.

Like a painting, your back is delicate. Back pain is the leading cause of disability among men under 45, and 80 percent of all people eventually get it. By building up your back in the weight room, you get a two-fold payoff: You'll stave off the injuries of tomorrow and construct a masterpiece of muscle today.

Get Back

If the muscles in your back were indeed a painting, the central images would be the *latissimus dorsi*, the *rhomboideus* and the *erector*

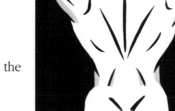

spinae. The background and foreground would be the smaller, supporting muscles deep beneath the skin's surface, and the shading and other detail would be the 24 movable vertebrae, the intervertebral disks and their connecting nerves and ligaments. Together, these components play a huge role in everything you do, from swinging a golf club to picking weeds.

The *latissimus dorsi*, or lats, run along your sides. Properly developed, they give your upper body that V-shaped look every guy wants. They extend, rotate and pull your arms toward your body. They also help you cough.

The *rhomboideus* include the rhomboideus major and minor, but are called the rhomboids for short. They're compact muscles located a few inches down from your neck, between your spine and shoulder blades. Their job is to retract and rotate your shoulder blades.

The *erector spinae* run along your spine, which they help support and move. The erector spinae are actually three distinct layers of muscle, the iliocostalis, the longissimus and the spinalis. Together they're responsible for extending your spine and flexing it to either side.

Here's how to get back to your future.

Lats
One-Arm Dumbbell Rows

Stand partly over a bench, with your body weight resting on your bent left leg and left hand, both of which should be on the center of the padded portion of the bench. With your right foot firmly on the floor, hold a dumbbell in your right hand. Keep your back straight, eyes facing the ground. Extend your right arm down toward the ground, elbow unlocked.

Pull the weight up and in toward your torso. Raise it as high as you can, bringing it into your lower chest muscles. Your right elbow should be pointing up toward the ceiling as you lift. Lower. When finished with the right side, reverse position and work the left arm.

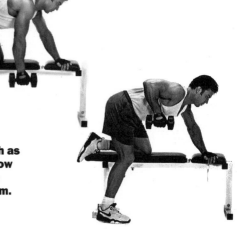

Lower Back
Stiff-Legged Dumbbell Deadlifts

Stand upright holding two light dumbbells in front of you with a palms-down grip. With the dumbbell handles each about shoulder-width apart, bend over at the waist, keeping your back straight. Keep your legs stiff, but knees unlocked, and your arms hanging down, but elbows unlocked.

Lift the dumbbells by raising your torso to the upright position. Keep your back, arms and legs straight, but don't lock your knees or elbows. Lift the dumbbells as if you're standing up. They should be at about upper-thigh level when done. Lower.

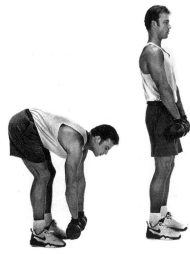

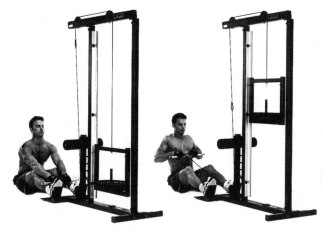

Lats and Upper Back
Seated Pulley Rows

Sit in a pulley row machine, grasping the handle in a narrow grip. Anchor your feet against the foot pedals, with your knees slightly bent and upper body upright, with a slight forward lean. Stretch your arms as far forward as you can while still maintaining your grip and proper technique.

Pull the handle of the machine in toward your body until it touches your lower chest. Keep your torso upright, legs fully extended (but not locked) and elbows pointing behind you. Lower.

Lats
Lat Pull-Downs

Sit at a lat pull-down machine. (Unless it doesn't have a seat, in which case kneel underneath it.) Grasp the handle overhead with as wide a grip as is comfortable, or at least wider than shoulder-width. Palms are facing away from your body, upper body is straight, eyes forward.

Pull the bar down to your body, behind your neck. Your upper body stays in the same upright position, but your elbows should be pointing at the ground and slightly outward. Raise to the starting position.

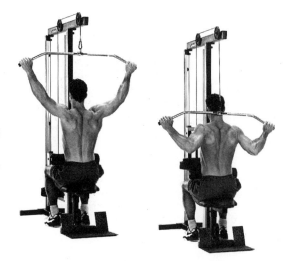

Lower Back
Good-Morning Exercise

Stand with your legs shoulder-width apart, holding a barbell with very light weights across your shoulders and behind your neck. Your hands should be a little wider apart than your shoulders, with palms facing out. Keep your upper body upright, shoulders back, chest out, and lower back straight with a slight forward lean.

Keeping your back level, slowly bend over at the waist until your body is roughly at a 90-degree angle and parallel to the floor. Keep your head up and back straight. Keep your legs straight and knees unlocked. Raise to the starting position.

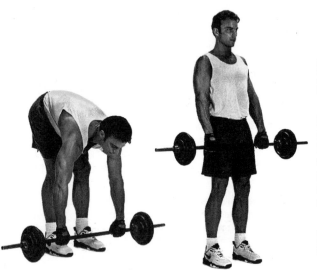

Lower Back
Stiff-Legged Deadlifts

Stand upright with a lightly weighted barbell in front of you. Keeping your back straight, bend over the barbell and grasp it with both hands, palms down, in a medium grip shoulder-width apart. Keep your legs stiff, but make sure your knees are unlocked and very slightly flexed. Keep your arms straight and elbows unlocked.

Lift the barbell to upper-thigh level. Your back, arms and legs stay straight. Keep your knees unlocked. Lower.

Lats and Upper Back
Bent-Over Rows

Stand bent over at the waist, back straight, hands gripping a barbell palms down in a wide grip. Feet are shoulder-width apart, neck straight, face pointing toward the floor. Keep your legs straight and knees unlocked.

Keeping your back straight, pull the barbell in toward your body so the bar is touching your lower chest. Your elbows should be pointing up toward the ceiling. Lower.

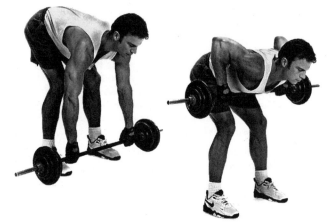

Lower Back
Back Extensions

Position yourself in a back extension machine, ankles locked behind the padded bars, groin area and upper thighs resting on the padded platform. Your hips should be over the edge of the platform, and your body bent over until your back is parallel to the floor. Fold your arms across your chest.

Bend over at the waist, with your upper torso lowered to the point where it's just a few inches above being perpendicular to the floor. Your arms should still be crossed over your chest and the rest of your body should stay in the starting position. Raise to the starting position.

The ⬆ next level

Upper Back: **T-Rows**

Straddle a T-bar rowing machine with your feet firmly on the ground. Using a narrow grip, hold the T-bar slightly off the ground so your back is relatively straight and not hunched. Bend your legs slightly and keep your upper body as straight as possible, but bent over at the waist.

Lift the T-bar up toward your body as you would in a normal bent-over row. Bring the weight up as high as you can, or until it touches your lower chest. There will be a little more up-and-down movement of your upper body, but don't sway or rock to gain momentum. Your elbows should be pointing up and slightly out as you lift. Lower.

Lower Back: **Back Extensions with Weights**

Do a back extension with proper technique, but hold a weight plate to your chest with your arms crossed over it. Start with light weight, then add more as your muscles get stronger.

Shoulders and Neck

It's easy to admire the posture of military men. They carry themselves with an alert energy, like peacocks in uniform.

"There's something about standing tall with your shoulders back and your chest out that says power," says Larry Brown, a retired U.S. Army and Air Force sergeant living in New Tripoli, Pennsylvania.

One way of getting this power-posture—short of six weeks' basic training—is to build the muscles in your shoulders, chest and arms, says Creighton University's Dr. Thomas R. Baechle.

"Your upper-body development affects your image," he says. "When you walk into a room, you command respect by the way you carry yourself. You don't want to look like you're peeping down a deep hole."

Shoulders to Show Off

Your shoulder muscles are called the deltoids. The name is descriptive, deriving

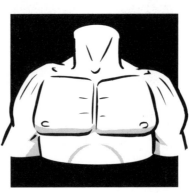

from the Latin word for "triangular in outline." The deltoid arises from various surfaces on your collarbone and shoulder blades and is connected to your humerus, the large bone in your upper arm. It lifts, rotates and extends your arm. Weight lifters talk about the anterior, lateral and posterior parts of the delts, meaning the front, side and back "heads" of the muscle. Each gets specific attention from various exercises for a well-rounded appearance. For example, side lateral raises work the sides of your deltoids; front raises mostly work the fronts.

As far as your neck goes, the only real muscle you need to know is the *trapezius*. It slopes down the sides of your neck, from the base of the skull to the middle of your back. The trapezius raises your shoulders and rotates your shoulder blades.

While working your shoulders, don't be discouraged if you tire halfway through your second set. "The shoulder muscles are not designed for endurance; they're designed for strength. If you've ever tried painting a ceiling with a paint roller, you know it doesn't take long before your shoulders wear out," says Dr. James E. Graves of the Department of Health and Education at Syracuse University.

Trapezius
Shoulder Shrugs

Standing upright, hold a lightly weighted barbell across your thighs using a medium grip, palms in toward your body. Feet are shoulder-width apart, with shoulders back but drooped down as far as they naturally will go. Chest is out and lower back is straight, with a slight forward lean.

Lift the barbell up and out by raising both shoulders to the front of your body. At the highest point, rotate your shoulders toward your ears, lifting them higher. Lower.

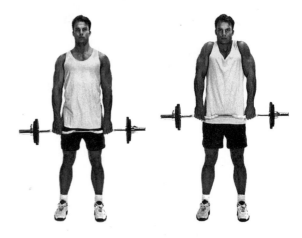

Deltoids
Seated Military Presses

Straddle the end of a bench with your feet a little farther than shoulder-width apart. Hold a barbell across the front of your shoulders with palms facing out, hands shoulder-width apart and elbows pointing down. Your back should be perpendicular to the ground, with shoulders back, chest out and lower back slightly leaning forward.

Lift the barbell above your head until your arms are fully extended. Don't lock your elbows, and don't sway or rock your body to gain momentum. Lower.

Note: Wear a weight belt for this exercise to support your lower back.

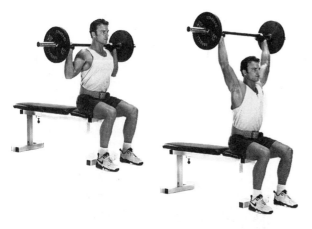

Deltoids
Behind-the-Neck Presses

Straddle the end of a bench with your feet a little farther than shoulder-width apart. Hold a barbell behind your neck and across your deltoids and trapezius with palms out, hands shoulder-width apart and elbows pointing down. Your back should be perpendicular to the ground, with shoulders back, chest out and a slight forward lean to your lower back.

Lift the barbell above your head, arms fully extended, elbows unlocked. Don't sway or arch your upper body for momentum. Lower.

Note: Wear a weight belt for this exercise to support your lower back.

Deltoids, Trapezius
Upright Rows

Stand upright holding a barbell in both hands, palms facing in toward your body in a narrow grip, hands a few inches from the center of the barbell. Arms are fully extended down in front of you, and the barbell is at upper-thigh level. Shoulders are slightly drooped forward, but your back is erect with a slight forward lean in the lower back.

Lift the barbell up, pulling it toward your head until it's under your chin. Your elbows should be pointing out. Don't sway or rock for momentum. Hold, lower.

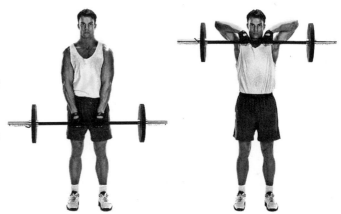

Lateral Deltoids
Side Lateral Raises

Stand upright, arms at your sides, holding a dumbbell in each hand, with palms facing toward your body and elbows slightly bent. Keep your shoulders back, chest out and lower back straight with a slight forward lean. Feet are shoulder-width apart.

Raise both dumbbells in unison in a straight line until they're shoulder level. Make sure your elbows are slightly bent, and keep your arms in the same plane as your torso. Lower.

Anterior Deltoids
Alternating Front Lateral Raises

Stand upright with your arms in front holding a dumbbell in each hand, palms facing your body and elbows slightly bent. Shoulders are back, chest out and lower back straight with a slight forward lean. Feet are shoulder-width apart.

Raise one dumbbell toward the ceiling until it's shoulder level. Don't lock your elbow. Lower, raise the other arm. Repeat, alternating your reps.

Note: You also can do this exercise with both hands using a lightly weighted barbell. Just don't sway your body and be sure to wear a weight belt for support.

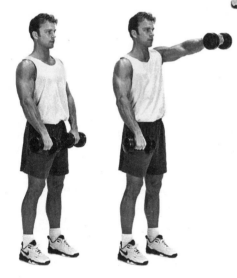

Posterior Deltoids
Bent-Over Lateral Raises

Bend over at the waist, a dumbbell in each hand. Palms face in toward each other, and arms are before you, elbows slightly bent. Feet are slightly wider than shoulder-width, and your back is straight and roughly parallel to the floor.

Raise dumbbells in unison out toward your sides as if you were flapping your arms. Raise your arms until they're parallel to the floor. Keep your back straight. Lower.

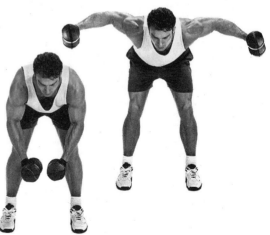

Deltoids
Alternating Seated Dumbbell Presses

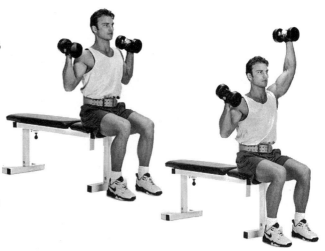

Grasp two dumbbells and straddle a bench with your legs slightly parted, feet firmly on the floor and arms raised. Hold the dumbbells about shoulder-width apart at shoulder level, palms facing each other. Shoulders are back, chest out and lower back slightly forward.

Raise the left dumbbell up until your arm is straight, but don't lock your elbow. Lower, repeat with the other arm. Repeat, alternating your reps.

***Note:* Wear a weight belt for this exercise to support your lower back.**

The 🔼 next level

Deltoids: Vertical Push-Ups

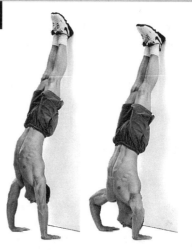

Get in a handstand position with your back toward a wall. Hands are shoulder-width or slightly wider apart, whichever's more comfortable. Legs are together or slightly apart, whichever helps you keep your balance. A partner can help by holding your legs.

Bend your arms, lowering yourself to the ground as far as you can go. Try to touch your head to the floor. If you can go lower, touch your nose or chin to the floor. Raise to the starting position.

Note: Use a spotter for this exercise.

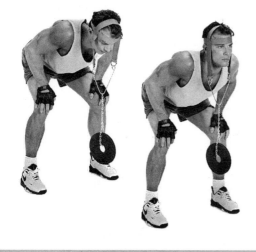

Neck Muscles: Neck Extensions

Strap on a neck extension headpiece with light weights hanging from the other end. Bend over at the waist so the weights are dangling before you. Rest your hands on your thighs. Keep your back straight, but bend over until your torso is roughly parallel to the floor.

Raise your head as far as it will go comfortably. The rest of your body stays in the starting position. Lower your head, moving only your neck.

Note: Start using light weights for this exercise, since it works your neck muscles more than usual.

Hands, Wrists and Forearms

While a chiseled chest may epitomize power for most guys, those muscles aren't used nearly as often as the ones in your hands and forearms. Think about it: Every time you make a fist, turn a doorknob, open a jar or wave good-bye, you're using the muscles in your hands, wrists and forearms.

"People probably think more about exercising their upper arms, but you need to spend some time on your lower arms, too," says Chip Harrison, strength and conditioning coach at Pennsylvania State University in State College. "A good exercise that works your grip will work the muscles in your hands and forearms."

Once you've enhanced your forearm and grip strength, you'll be more handy throwing a ball or swinging a bat, Harrison says. To prove it, Penn State had its college softball players perform forearm and grip strengthening exercises in a study. The result was a 12 to 15 percent average increase in strength. And although that improved strength doesn't necessarily translate into better batting averages, Harrison explains, the players are now able to train harder and put more stress on those muscles when they're throwing a ball or swinging a bat.

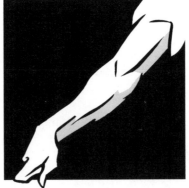

Armed and Dangerous

When you're talking power of the hands and wrists, you're really talking forearms. Also called the antebrachium, your forearms are the meaty section of your arm between your wrist and elbow.

Your forearms control most of your gross gripping strength during activities that don't require fine motor skills, like swinging a golf club. In comparison, activities that require fine motor skills, like painting a model airplane or playing the piano, require a combination of forearm muscles and the smaller muscles in your hands.

The forearms are home to three main muscle groups: the *brachioradialis*, the *flexors* and the *extensors*. The brachioradialis runs from your humerus, the large bone in your upper arm, to the lower end of your radius, the bone on the thumb-side of your forearm.

The names of the specific flexors and extensors in your forearm read like entries in a Latin dictionary. All you really need to know is that the flexors move your palm toward your forearm. Some of the flexors also help move your fingers.

The extensors move the back of your hand toward your forearm and also help extend your fingers.

Here are some routines you can do to give your forearms that pumped-up Popeye look.

Forearms, Hand
Grippers

Select a gripper device that offers moderate resistance and squeeze it closed. Release and repeat. Go for the most reps possible, then switch hands. Try this exercise while watching television or talking on the phone. You can do this anywhere, anytime, for a fast, effective hand workout.

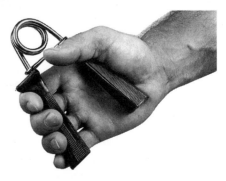

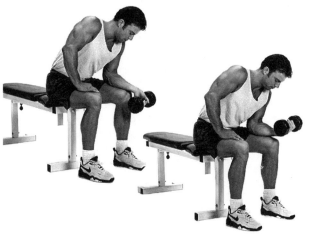

Forearm Flexors, Wrists
Forearm Curls

Sit at the end of a bench with your legs slightly wider than hip-width apart. Your right hand should be on your right thigh, and you should be holding a dumbbell in your left hand, with a palm-up grip. Your left wrist should be slightly over your left knee, so you can bend your wrist through its full range of motion. The top of your forearm should be resting against your thigh, and your upper body should be upright, but you may lean slightly into your left leg for comfort.

Curl the dumbbell in a semicircular motion up toward your body as far as you can. Don't let your arm rise up off your thigh. At the top of the curl, hold for a second, then lower to the starting position. Finish your reps, then switch hands.

Note: This also can be done with both hands and a barbell.

Forearm Extensors, Wrists
Reverse Forearm Curls

Sit at the end of a bench with your legs slightly wider than hip-width apart. Your left hand should be on your left thigh, and you should be holding a dumbbell in your right hand, with a palm-down grip. Your wrist should be slightly over your knee, so that you're able to bend it through its full range of motion. The bottom, meaty part of your forearm should be resting against your thigh, and your upper body should be fairly upright, but you may lean slightly into your right leg for comfort.

Curl the dumbbell in a semicircular motion up toward your body as far as you can. Don't let your arm rise up off your thigh. At the top of the curl, hold for a second, then lower to the starting position. Finish your reps, then switch hands.

Note: Use a lighter weight for this than you would for a normal forearm curl.

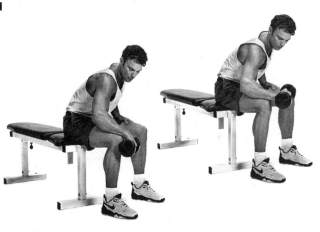

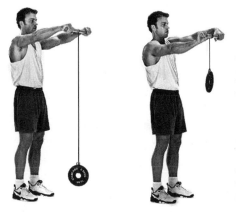

Forearms, Wrists
Wrist Rollers

Stand upright, feet about shoulder-width apart, holding the wrist roller in both hands, palms down, with your arms extended in front of you. The weight should be dangling in front of you.

Slowly roll the weight up with your wrists, using long exaggerated up-and-down movements with your wrists to get their full range of motion. Keep the rest of your body stationary—don't sway your body or drop your arms. When the weight has reached the top, slowly lower it using the same motion.

Feet and Ankles

What's one of the most important body parts involved in a punch?

Shoulders? Knuckles? Good try. But you're overlooking something—literally. According to Joe Lewis—a guy who knows punching like Jimmy Buffett knows margaritas—it's your feet and ankles.

"The power in your punch comes from the power in your ankles," says Lewis, a former amateur world karate champ who trained with Bruce Lee and has been called the greatest karate fighter of all time. "When you throw a punch, what you're really doing is firing that punch with your feet and ankles."

Of course, the importance of your feet and ankles doesn't stop there. On an average day these underdogs of your anatomy carry around the equivalent of 200 tons of weight. When you're running, each foot braves a buffeting 500 pounds of pressure with every step you take.

Get on the Sole Train

Your feet and ankles are structural marvels, remarkably well-adapted to the vital role they play in keeping you moving. Each foot has 26 bones, though some people are

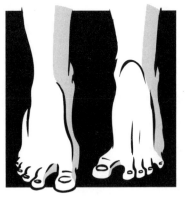

born with a few more or less. There are more than 100 ligaments in each foot and 33 muscles, some of which are attached to your lower leg. Your feet also are the anchoring point for the biggest tendon in your body: the Achilles tendon, a fibrous rope that attaches your calf muscles to your heel bone.

Three sections comprise each foot: the *tarsals* (the bones of the rear foot), the *metatarsals* (the bones of the mid-foot) and the *phalanges* (the toe bones). The toes help you push off with every step, and the heel pad and arch of your foot act as shock absorbers when you land.

Perhaps the most important muscles concerning your feet and ankles—and by far the easiest to work in the weight room—are your calf muscles (the *gastrocnemius* and *soleus*) and their counterparts, the *anterior tibial* muscles, which run along your shin. The gastrocs and soleus give your calves that well-rounded athletic look. They help you run and jump by flexing your foot downward. The tibs do the same, except they flex your foot up.

Granted, feet and ankles get exercise enough shuffling you through the day, but if you have the time—or if you have ambitions of competing in any sport—it pays to give these guys a workout once in a while.

Here's how to work the muscles that will keep your feet and ankles strong.

Feet Muscles
Towel Crunches

Take off your shoes and sit on a chair. Spread a towel across the floor and, grasping one end with your toes, crunch it under your feet. Use the muscles in the bottom of your feet and in your toes. Keep your heel on the floor at all times.

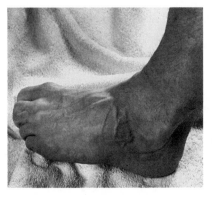

Anterior Tibialis
Weighted Foot Flexes

Sit on a table so your feet are dangling in the air. You should be wearing ankle weights wrapped around your feet, near the base of your toes. Your upper body should be upright, arms resting at your sides, and your toes should be pointing down to the floor in a natural, unflexed position.

Raise your toes up toward your shins as high as possible. The rest of your body should stay the same, but your weighted toes should be lifted up and in, so you feel the contraction in the muscles along your shin. Return to the starting position.

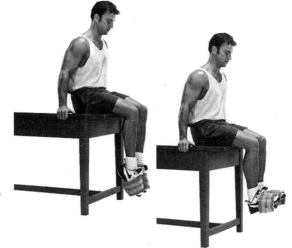

Anterior Tibialis
Toe Raises

Stand upright with your toes over the ledge of a weight plate or staircase step. Hold on to a wall with one hand for balance, if you need to. Your toes should be extended as far out over the edge as you can, but maintain your posture and balance and keep your heels on the floor.

Pull your toes in toward your shins as far as you can. The rest of your body should remain upright, and you should feel the contraction around your shins. Hold for a second, then lower.

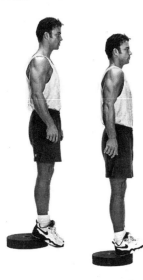

Anterior Tibialis
Bowlegged Toe Raises

Do toe raises as you normally would, but start with your toes splayed outward with your body weight focused on the outsides of your feet in a bowlegged position. This stresses the muscles slightly differently than in the standard position.

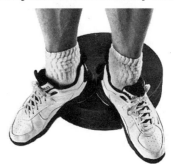

Anterior Tibialis
Knock-Kneed Toe Raises

Do standard toe raises as you normally would, but start with your toes splayed inward with your body weight focused on the insides of your feet in a knock-kneed position. This will stress the muscles slightly differently than in the standard position.

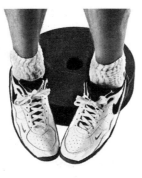

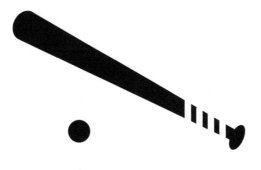

Part Three

Power at Play

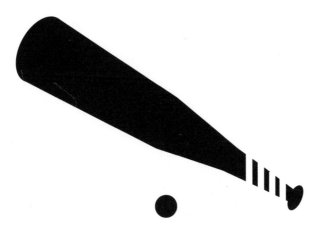

Running

Distance Makes the Legs Grow Stronger

As though evidence were really needed that your local pub might not be the best place to do your resistance training, we present Exhibit A: bungee running.

In a new variation of the old carrot-and-stick motivational method, someone in England came up with the bright idea of combining running, drinking and bungee jumping. ("Gee, why didn't I think of that?" you're no doubt thinking.) As crowds madly cheer them on, pubgoers strap themselves to a bungee cord, run so it stretches to its limit and grab a pint of beer. If they're lucky, they may even get a sip before they are sent hurtling back, arse over head. If they're unlucky, they get hurt or—as happened to one 35-year-old contestant on the Isle of Man—die of brain injuries.

In an example of typical British understatement, researchers examining this fad concluded: "Perhaps when played in pubs, the participants may be less in control of their minds and movements than this sport demands."

No kidding. Here's some simple advice: Have a beer in the pub. Save your resistance training for the gym.

Running Strong, Running Long

There definitely is a role for resistance training in running. Just forget about the bungee cord. Weight lifting can make you a stronger runner.

But there is an even more compelling reason to incorporate resistance training into your workout regimen: It can keep you running longer.

"Weight lifting can reduce injuries," says U.S. marathoner Steve Spence, who captured a bronze medal at the 1991 World Championships in Tokyo. "And anyone can benefit from that."

Spence, of Chambersburg, Pennsylvania, is one of the new breed of runners who regularly uses weight training to enhance performance. For years runners were told that if they wanted to run faster, they simply had to run. To a degree, that still holds true. "The most important thing is to run if you want to become a better runner," Spence says.

But resistance training, coupled with daily stretching to increase flexibility, "allows you to stay injury-free," says Budd Coates, a national-class distance runner and *Men's Health* magazine fitness consultant. "Strength training alone won't make you a better runner. It's an effective supplement, but it can't be the focus."

That's an important point. Recreational runners shouldn't think they can substitute a weight-lifting workout for running, and then run faster on the roads. "Most people have an energy pie. And they only have a limited time for running," Spence says. So don't subtract from your running time to add a weight workout.

However, if you can make the time to add a couple of weight-lifting sessions to your weekly workouts, you'll find that you can stay on the roads longer—and run faster.

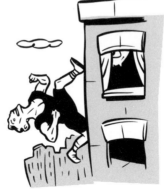

Weight Gains

While some experts maintain that your legs get all the strengthening they need from running, Coates says weight training can help correct the natural imbalance running creates between the hamstrings and the quadriceps muscles. Distance running builds stronger hamstrings than quads. Working both muscle groups with weights—at a three-to-two ratio favoring the quads—will keep them in sync, Coates says.

He recommends leg extensions for the quads, and leg curls for the hamstrings. If you work with 30 pounds on leg extensions, use no more than 20 pounds for the leg curls.

Those who say weight lifting won't directly make you run faster are right, Coates says. But they're missing the point. By strengthening your legs and correcting muscle imbalances that could result in injuries to your legs or lower back, weight lifting "allows you to do the kind of running that will decrease your 5-K time."

It's also critical to build strong postural muscles—those that help you remain upright. That means your abdomen, lower back, upper back, shoulders and neck. "When you start to lose your form, usually it's the posture that goes," Spence says. "Once you start to lose it in a race and start to fatigue, you can never really get it back."

Jeff Galloway, a former U.S. Olympic marathoner who has worked with thousands of runners and authored the best-selling *Galloway's Book on Running*, says strengthening your postural muscles delivers a three-way payoff: "They tend to keep you upright longer, which makes you more efficient; reduce injuries and make you feel better when you run."

It's important to maintain an upright position while running because that keeps the chest cavity open, allowing the lungs to take in more air. "It's a numbers game," says Galloway. "You get more oxygen into the right places at the

---

Power ⬆ Tip

Like most runners, world-class marathoner Steve Spence doesn't like to spend a lot of time in the gym.

"I like to get in and out in a half hour, so I try to make efficient use of that time," Spence says. During the winter, when his mileage increases and intensity declines, Spence is in the gym five or six days a week. He works his upper body and lower body on alternating days, doing a circuit-type routine with only about 30 seconds of rest between sets.

He'll do a total of two to three sets with 10 to 12 repetitions for each exercise. "If I'm doing three upper-body exercises, I'll just circuit them until I do three sets so I don't have much downtime," Spence says. "It's not really an aerobic workout. I'm not breathing heavy or anything. It's just so I don't have the downtime."

When spring arrives, Spence cuts back to two days a week, doing only one or two sets for each exercise. And once the racing season arrives, he sets the weights aside. But he doesn't give up resistance training.

"I do push-ups and crunches year-round," Spence says. "I like doing them at night. If I'm watching TV for an hour, I'll do push-ups and sit-ups during commercials. And that's pretty much a year-round thing for me, and almost every day."

---

right time, and there's more oxygen absorption."

Galloway, speaking "as one runner to another," personally favors crunches, back extensions, upright rows and shoulder shrugs to build strength in the postural muscles.

Coates adds that doing push-ups through the full range of motion will help stretch the chest. And doing lateral raises and biceps curls will help build stronger arms and shoulders, allowing you to hold your arms in proper form during long runs.

Head for the Hills

If you love to run but aren't that crazy about the gym, there's good news: You can still do resistance training.

"I definitely believe in resistance work that's done in the running motion. For instance: hill training or sand training," Galloway says. "I think those two are extremely beneficial for running. The bottom line is that running is not a strength activity. We're not trying to overcome gravity. We're trying to defy it.

"However, there is a definite advantage in having strategic running muscle groups strengthened a little bit more than they need to be strengthened, just so they can overcome extreme usage, push beyond current limits and avoid injury," he says.

Galloway says you can get injury-prevention protection and build strength by incorporating long and short hills into your training.

Galloway defines a short hill as any incline of one-quarter mile or less. Running hard—slightly faster than your 5-K pace—on short hills helps build explosive power. One word of caution, though: "Never sprint, because sprinting up a hill or down a hill can really lead to injury quickly," Galloway says.

Longer hills are in the one-half mile to mile range. "I'd certainly not recommend anything more than a mile," Galloway says. Running long hills at your 10-K pace builds endurance strength. "The way you work on speed and technique on the hill is not through longer stride length, but through quicker turnover rate," Galloway says. "In other words, you keep

Using Reverse Psychology

Timothy "Bud" Badyna has made a career out of running backwards. He comes by his power, well, straightforwardly.

Badyna, who is in his late twenties, holds three titles in the Guinness Book of World Records: for running a 5-K race backwards in 21 minutes, 50 seconds; a 10-K race backwards in 45 minutes, 37 seconds and a marathon backwards in 3 hours, 53 minutes, 17 seconds.

While it may look odd, retro-running—as it is called by proponents—offers numerous health and fitness benefits. Studies have shown it burns one-third more calories (about 130 calories per mile for the average male, as opposed to 100 for running), elevates the heart rate more effectively (173 beats per minute in reverse compared to 149 forward) and demands greater oxygen consumption.

As Badyna looks back on his triumphs, the six-foot-two Atlanta paramedic identifies these winning strategies.

Get pumped. When he's working up to a big race, Ba-

shortening your stride as the grade of the hill gets steeper."

He recommends starting with 4 hill repeats and gradually increasing by 1 a week until you can run 8 to 12. Jog down slowly to recover between repeats, and always give yourself at least two days rest between hill workouts.

If you're a flatlander, don't fear. Parking garage inclines, stadium steps, office building stairs and treadmills with hill settings can all do the trick. But a more scenic alternative is to hit the beach.

Running in the sand provides the same benefits and follows the same basic guidelines, Galloway says. You can do short runs at a quicker pace or longer runs at a more moderate dyna hits the Nautilus machines three or four times a week for total-body resistance training and runs six or seven times a week. While quadriceps and calf muscles are crucial to backwards running, his legs get no extra attention in the weight room beyond routine leg curls and extensions.

Toss out the junk. Even when he's not in training, Badyna says, he's blessed with a "killer metabolism" that flames away burgers and cupcakes before they can make the slightest blip on his lean frame. Even so, when he's getting ready to back into a marathon, he eschews all junk food and alcohol and favors juices and sports drinks.

Cover your rear. What works with free weights applies to backwards running, too: Use a spotter to keep you out of trouble. "With my first three world records I basically used a spotter the whole time, somebody riding a bicycle behind me. Actually *in front* of me. Well, we were facing each other. Cars give you a little bit more room when you have a bicyclist with you."

Stretching for the Long Run

Steve Spence may be a world-class runner, but when it comes to stretching, he's just like you. "I don't think anybody really likes to stretch. It's something that needs to be done," he says.

Spence listens to his body, stretching for about ten minutes before his first workout of the day and then doing lighter stretching before later workouts. He also does light massage and stretching following a run. "The main thing you want to do is a good hamstring stretch and a good quad stretch," Spence says. "If you're getting that in, it's pretty adequate."

It helps to loosen up before a run. But don't make the mistake of rolling out of bed and trying to touch your toes. Do a light warm-up first—such as a few minutes of easy jogging—to get blood circulating to the muscles.

pace. There is one additional option: a long, gentle run, about once a week, alternating between loose sand and the firmer sand down by the waterline.

"Don't try to overload the muscles by running in loose sand for an extremely long distance," Galloway cautions. "It's sort of like running up a steep hill." In both cases—on steep hills or in loose sand—Galloway says runners should keep it short.

He advises starting with no more than 100 yards in loose sand, gradually working up to about 400 yards. "The long-term benefits are dramatic," Galloway says. "The give of sand provides a resistance that is even better than hills. But you really just have to watch it and make sure you don't turn an ankle in the process."

When it comes to which muscles you need to stretch, Budd Coates advises: "Listen to the squeaky wheel." Some of us are born with muscles more supple than others. If you're not one of the lucky ones, a little time stretching—no more than 15 minutes—can help keep you running injury-free.

So if a workout leaves your hamstrings doing their own rendition of the old Archie Bell and the Drells hit "Tighten Up," make sure you stretch. "The most beneficial time to stretch is after a workout," Coates says.

And that's especially true after a hard workout. If you're going to fudge on stretching, do it on your easy days—not when you're doing hill work or intervals on the track.

Coates offers a simple rule of thumb: "If you stress them, you'd better stretch them."

Bicycling

Power to the Pedal

If you came across a group of cyclists working out in the weight room, chances are you could make a fortune selling T-shirts that read: "I'd rather be riding."

Harvey Newton, an instructor at the University of Colorado at Colorado Springs who has worked with cyclists at the U.S. Olympic Training Center in Colorado Springs, Colorado, sympathizes with that sentiment. "The average cyclist is going to say, 'I don't want to be in the gym. I don't like it as much as being on the bike.' And that's certainly understandable," Newton says. "Given my druthers, in pleasant weather I'd rather be riding than be in the gym."

What cyclists need to understand, Newton says, is that the time they spend in the gym will keep them riding longer and more efficiently. It's not a matter of choosing one or the other.

"Nobody is going to get better on the bike by lifting weights solely. I think that's a really key point to make," says Newton, who also is director of program development for the National Strength and Conditioning Association. "Strength training has to be seen as supplemental to cycling."

That said, there is no question that lifting weights will help you lift your performance on the bike to new heights.

"Strength training will increase actual performance on the bike because strength is an important component of endurance," says Fred Matheny, fitness and training editor of *Bicycling* magazine and author of *Weight Training for Cyclists.* "The theory is that a stronger muscle uses fewer

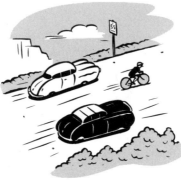

of its total muscle fibers in any given pedal stroke. So it fatigues less easily. The standard line is that you can't make a strong cyclist out of a weak person."

Stronger leg muscles will allow you to maintain your pedal cadence hour after hour. Instead of feeling fatigued halfway into a weekend 40-miler, you'll still feel fresh and strong because your muscles are working more efficiently. And, if you need a sudden burst of speed in the middle of a ride, weight lifting will help there, too.

Weight lifting doesn't just make you stronger on the bike. It makes you more powerful. "There's a difference between strength and power, with power being more explosive," Newton says.

Muscle and Myth

Many cyclists still fear that if they lift weights, they'll turn into the Incredible Bulk. As Daffy Duck might say, they're myth-taken.

"An awful lot of people have very bad information," Newton says. "They think if the weights are heavy, they're going to get big muscles. That's not the case."

Bulk primarily results from eating and genetics, experts say. "There is no exercise, there is no repetition system that makes you have a 19-inch arm. Otherwise, we'd all have them very easily," Newton says.

Cyclists often get the wrong idea because there is a natural tendency to gain weight during the off-season, when they concentrate most on weight lifting.

"The average cyclist should not fear gaining weight in the gym. It isn't going to happen, unless they're eating more and riding less," Newton says. "And at holiday time, which is when most people, unfortunately, are strength training, they *are* riding less and they *are* eating more. Then they say, 'Oh no, I've gained ten pounds. It's the weights—I have to stop.' It has nothing to do with the weights."

Build a Balanced Body

To be a powerful cyclist, you need powerful legs. Specifically, the gluteal muscles, quadriceps and hamstrings are the keys to pedaling power.

Clearly, the more you ride, the more your legs are worked. That leads some cyclists—world-class riders as well as weekend tourers—to conclude they don't need to work their legs in the gym. Newton disagrees. "The fatigue factor involved with the average cyclist putting in *x* number of miles a week or a month is that they don't feel like going to the gym and working the legs," Newton says. "They'll either say that by working their legs, they are taking away from their riding, or by riding, they don't have the energy to work their legs. I think there are some ways to work around that. But so far, we haven't found too many takers."

Many cyclists who do leg exercises during the winter quit when the racing season rolls around. Newton, however, says cyclists would be better off cutting back—even to one day a week—to maintain the strength they've labored to build. "The legs are the prime movers, and we don't want to see any drop-off in strength there," he says.

Ed Burke, Ph.D., associate professor at the University of Colorado at Colorado Springs and vice-president of the National Strength and Conditioning Association, says the single best exercise for cyclists is the leg press. Squats, "when done properly," also help build the explosive power cycling demands, he says.

"Most of a cyclist's power comes from the hips down," Dr. Burke says. "I get nervous

---

Power ⬆ Tip

Squats are a favorite of many world-class cyclists, and for good reason: They work the gluteal muscles, quadriceps and hamstrings—all of which generate pedaling power.

World-champion sprint cyclist Marty Nothstein says technique is the key to getting the explosive power he needs from squats. "The old school was to use heavy weight, sit down low and push it up slowly," he says.

Going down too low places potentially dangerous strain on the knees, so Nothstein now squats only to a 90-degree angle—perpendicular to the floor. "He comes down slowly and actually stops," says his strength trainer, John Graham. But instead of slowly grunting the weight back up, Nothstein now comes out of the down position with what he calls "an explosive push."

"From a dead stop he explodes through the motion," Graham says. That simulates a similar explosive force required on the bike, when sprinting power is needed.

---

saying that because then people say, 'Oh, I don't need to do anything for my upper body.' But that's not true, either. The legs may provide most of the force, but you need to have an equal force above the waist to keep your seat in the saddle."

If you want the force to be with you, strengthening the muscles in your lower back, abdomen, shoulders and arms is essential.

"The key thing to remember is that cycling requires strength in muscles that it doesn't build strength in," Matheny says. "The abs are a really good example of that. You need really strong abdominals to protect your lower back and stabilize your pedaling stroke. But they never get really stressed when you're in a cycling position. So this supplemental work is crucial."

If you don't believe it, try this the next time you're out for a ride: As you pedal on a clear straightaway, reach back with one hand and feel the muscles in the small of your back. You'll find them contracting rhythmically to your pedal cadence.

"It's amazing, if you go out and do a lot of climbing on the bike, how tired your lower back gets," Matheny says. "It's pretty crucial to strengthen that up. That's where a lot of your back problems in cycling come from. It's not a disk problem. It's just fatigue in those muscles."

World-champion sprint cyclist Marty Nothstein, of Trexlertown, Pennsylvania, and his trainers call the abdominals and lower-back muscles "the pillars" of successful cycling. "A strong lower back and strong abdominals indirectly affect your leg workouts because you're putting a lot of weight on your back," Nothstein says. "You need something to support that. And not too many people realize that."

So experts recommend doing strengthening exercises for the abdominals and lower back. "Traditionally, cyclists have worked their abs but neglected their lower back," says Nothstein's strength coach John Graham, a certified strength and conditioning specialist and director of the Human Performance Center at the Allentown Sports Medicine and Human Performance Center in Allentown, Pennsylvania. "That creates a muscle imbalance. And if you injure your lower back, you're unable to compete."

Working your shoulders and arms is important because they have to carry roughly half your weight as you ride. Cycling doesn't build strong arms, but without them, you won't be able to ride for long. "The position you use to hold the handlebars requires that those muscles be strong," Graham says. "The rear shoulder is one of the most neglected muscles in cyclists."

A Plan for All Seasons

Strength training is a year-round process for cyclists who are serious about improving performance. But it doesn't have to be an ordeal. All you need is about 45 minutes to an hour, enough time to do five—count 'em, five—exercises.

During the off-season, aim for three workouts a week. When the pre-season rolls around, cut back to two, and once you're in the cycling season, one weight-lifting session a week will help you maintain the strength you've gained. Harvey Newton, director of program development for the National Strength and Conditioning Association, and Fred Matheny, fitness and training editor of *Bicycling* magazine, recommend a simplified routine that includes:

- An upper-body pushing exercise, such as a bench press or dips.
- An upper-body pulling exercise, such as rows or pull-ups.

Year-Round Power

Nothstein, who in 1994 became the first American cyclist ever to win two gold medals at the world championships, is often asked about his off-season routine. His answer is always the same: "I never have an off-season."

His training changes, with increased emphasis on weight lifting, "but I never let myself get out of shape," he says. "Most cyclists will say, 'It's wintertime. We don't have to train.' But I look at winter as a whole other season, and step it up as far as training goes."

One common mistake made by cyclists who do strength training in the off-season is to cut back drastically on their aerobic training. "I think it's really important that a cyclist not let his aerobic conditioning suffer in the off-season," Newton says. If you can't get outside on your bike during the winter, ride a stationary bike indoors, or spend time on a stair-climbing

- **An abdominal exercise, such as crunches.**
- **A lower-back exercise, such as back extensions.**
- **An exercise for the legs, such as leg presses or squats.**

For the first year of weight lifting, Newton advises doing three sets of ten repetitions for each of the five exercises. As you grow stronger, add weight. Working with the same weight over several months would be like always riding your bike in the same gear, on flat terrain, at the same pace over the same distance: You're never going to get any better.

Once you become more experienced, he recommends gradually increasing the weight even more, while lowering the number of repetitions in each set to five or six. That will provide you with maximum strength gains—which, after all, ought to be the goal of strength training.

Climb Every Mountain

Strength-training exercises are even more crucial for mountain bikers. Hurtling over rocks and flying down steep embankments not only is hard work but greatly increases your odds of crashing. A strong upper body may not guarantee that you will stay on your bike when you hit a rock, but it will increase your chances of not suffering a serious injury when you land.

With all the handling required in mountain biking, upper body strength takes on even greater importance than it does in road cycling. "In true mountain biking, one of the main concerns is the variation in terrain, the fact that you're frequently out of the saddle in a position where traction is not constant," Newton says. Pulling the front wheel over logs, hanging on during rough downhills and lugging your bike up unridable hills can add up to sore arm and shoulder muscles without proper conditioning.

"It's going to be most noticeable in the upper arms and upper back area," Newton says.

Upper-body pulling exercises—rows or pull-ups are two examples—can build the strength needed to pull on the handlebar to clear obstacles.

Plowing through mud and sand on a mountain bike certainly helps build strong legs, but weight lifting can give you a decided edge over those who get all of their strength on the bike.

There also is more of a strain on the midsection and lower back, as mountain bikers are constantly in and out of the saddle. You may not feel fatigued there as quickly as in the arms and shoulders, but paying attention to your abs and back will help keep you rolling long after the others have bit the dust.

machine, rowing machine or other aerobic exercise machine, he advises.

When cyclists who have lifted weights all winter quit once racing season arrives, it's like someone deciding to ride a bike to get in shape, doing it for three months and then stopping. "What happens? We go right back to where we were," says Newton, who has done two videotapes—*Strength Training for Cyclists: The Exercises* and *Strength Training for Cyclists: Program Planning*—demonstrating weight-lifting routines.

During the cycling season, which generally runs from May through September, leg strengthening exercises can be cut back—but not cut out entirely—because you'll be working your legs much harder on the bike.

"We cut back the volume," Graham says. "We won't train as often, and we'll do fewer sets and reps. But we'll train just as hard, intensity-wise. It's designed to maintain."

Wilderness Sports

Being Great Outdoors

When it comes to sports, there's no more challenging playing field than the one owned by Mother Nature. That's why so many men love outdoor activities—hiking, rock climbing, backpacking and fishing, to name some of the most popular. Scoring a touchdown or spiking the ball over the net simply pales in comparison to testing yourself against the raw power of the elements—it's about as good a challenge as you'll find on the planet. Add to that a huge visual and spiritual bonus—traveling through a landscape of pristine beauty and quiet serenity. But before you venture into the great outdoors, you'd be wise to remember the old Boy Scout motto: Be prepared.

"There's no question that one needs to do some type of physical training before heading out on the trail," says Byron Crouse, M.D., a physician in Duluth, Minnesota, who studied the health care needs of hikers on the Appalachian Trail. The problem is that so few people adequately train indoors for strenuous activity in the great outdoors. During his research Dr. Crouse found that at least 30 percent of hikers suffered some type of injury during the course of a trip, many of which he says could have been prevented by pre-training.

"Of course, there's always a possibility of injury when you're in the outdoors, and no amount of exercise beforehand may prevent it," says Dr. Crouse. "But I believe many basic muscle injuries can be reduced or eliminated if people take the time to train a few months—or even a few weeks—before they

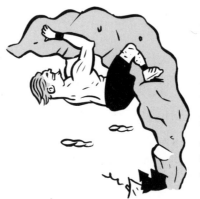

go out into the wilderness." Dr. Crouse's message is as clear as a mountain stream—before you hit the trail, hit the gym.

Walk on the Wild Side

If you want to scale that mountain or land that prize salmon, chances are your sport utility vehicle won't take you all the way—at some point, you'll have to get out and hoof it. And if you're backpacking, walking will be your main activity. That's good: Brisk walking on a regular street or sidewalk is already recommended by exercise experts as a great aerobic and cardiovascular workout. Walking on a trail with 50 pounds of gear lashed to your back is that much better—not only are you working out your legs and back, you're building your heart and lungs to a phenomenal degree.

But like a lot of strenuous pastimes, you get the most benefit out of hiking by preparing for it with a formal weight-training workout that ensures you won't injure yourself. Bearing that in mind, Dr. Crouse says outdoorsmen should devote extra attention to the areas they use and abuse the most—the upper and lower back, abdominals, thighs and calves.

Here are some basic tips to help prepare you for a wild time.

Pack a rope. One of the easiest—but best—leg exercises, jumping rope improves coordination as well as muscular ability. "Ten minutes with a jump rope just works wonders," says David Lillard, president of the American Hiking Society in Washington, D.C. "If you're backpacking and carrying 45 to 65 pounds on your back and going up a steep slope, you'll need leg and back strength to push you forward." In addition to jumping rope, lower-body strength training and abdominal and lower-back exercises will give you that.

Take the stairs. Stair-climbing builds explosive power in the legs and helps strengthen the knees, too. "If you work in an office or live in an apartment building with only three or four floors, there's no excuse—you should never use the elevator," Lillard says. If your building is several stories tall, take the stairs at least once a day.

Shop with your pack. Lillard says a personal favorite training tactic is to load a pack and walk around the neighborhood a few times in the days before a trip. "We also have a guy here in the office who doesn't use a cart when he goes shopping—he just loads everything into his backpack," says Lillard. Hint: Let the store manager in on your little training secret, unless you want to carry a shoplifting rap, too.

Park and walk. "Make it a game to park your car far away from where you're going—the mall, the office—and walk on in," says Lillard.

Break in your boots. As a matter of common sense, if you've bought new hiking boots, you should spend several weeks breaking them in. "You'd be surprised how many people ignore common sense and buy new boots the day before they hit the trail," says Dr. Crouse. Besides the fact that this will cause blisters and can leave you prone to other injuries, wearing boots only a day before you head out doesn't give your body time to adjust.

"Even if you have well-worn boots, I suggest walking around in them every day for a couple of weeks before you go on a trip," Lillard says. This gets your body and your sense of balance used to the extra weight and tread of a hiking boot.

The Wilderness Workout

Besides sports-specific exercises, you can modify your regular fitness and weight-training workout in order to beef up the muscles you'll

---

Power ⬆ Tip

When it comes to hiking, if you have a friend in knees, you have a friend, indeed. "Some people have to give up hiking or strenuous backpacking because their knees can't take it. They just blow out," says David Lillard, president of the American Hiking Society. "I think that focusing on the knee—keeping it strong with exercises off the trail—will be the factor that enables you to stay on the trail."

Most hikers love to do other outdoor sports, Lillard says. Cycling, running, cross-country skiing and snowshoeing are the most popular. "And these are great training exercises, too, because they work your leg and lower-back muscles, which are essential," Lillard says. "Plus, these sports strengthen the muscles around the knee, which is probably the most important thing you can do. Out on the trail, nothing takes punishment like the knee."

Need we say more?

---

need in the backcountry.

"Working out year-round—lifting weights, doing cardiovascular work—in preparation for wilderness activities is not simply helpful, it's really very smart. In fact, it might save your life," Dr. Crouse says. Next time you hit the health club, work these exercises into your routine so you can literally be a mountain man.

Be wild at heart. Most health clubs are bristling with strength-training and exercise equipment that will work the muscles you use in the great outdoors. "And they can train your heart and lungs, which will give you more power and endurance when you're on the trail hauling 40 or 50 pounds of gear on your back," Lillard says. This equipment includes free weights, resistance machines, stair-climbers, stationary cycles and cross-country skiers. "Some clubs have a machine called a mountain-climber," says Lillard. The device has steps like a stair-climbing machine, as well as handles that move in time to the stair-steps. "Your arms and legs are moving at the same time, and let me tell you: It's an exhausting workout," he says.

Be flexible. Flexibility is key in the backcountry. Pounding over rocks, climbing up escarpments—you'll need strong and supple muscles to take the punishment, particularly in the thighs. "Your quads and hamstrings are going to take a beating out there," Lillard says. But you can limber them up with a series of quadriceps, hamstring and hip and lower-leg stretches, says certified strength and conditioning specialist John Graham.

Build a strong back. A well-made backpack balances the weight through your hips, back and shoulders. Still, since your back is taking the place of a pack-mule, you want to make sure it's going to be ready for hours of hauling your gear. Before you go—and before you cinch up your pack every day on the trail—take a few minutes to do a back flexion by lying flat on your back, grasping your legs under the knees and pulling your knees toward your chest. Then, do some back extensions—lie on your stomach, keeping your back relaxed. With your fingers cupped behind your ears, raise your shoulders slightly, but keep your pelvis against the floor.

Lunge into the wilds. During your normal weight-training routine, be sure to spend some time strengthening the thigh muscles. You can do that best with squats and front lunges. As you do them, be sure to keep your back and neck straight. Do at least three sets of each exercise, and 10 to 12 repetitions per set.

Go for your gut. The upper and lower abdominals support your back and, therefore, much of your pack. To strengthen them, do a

variety of crunches. In addition to the traditional crunch, do some raised-leg crunches as well. Finally, to work the oblique muscles on your sides, do a normal crunch, then twist slightly toward your left knee as you raise up. Lower yourself back to the floor, then raise again and twist slightly to your right knee.

Shoulder the burden. In addition to your back, your shoulder and neck muscles may feel some strain after hauling a pack or clambering up a cliff face. Shoulder shrugs are a great shoulder and neck trainer, as is the upright row.

One final note: Once you've prepared your body, don't blow it all by failing to properly prepare for your trip. Just as you

Fishing for Fitness

Although you need to be in good hiking trim to reach some of the best fishing spots, once you get there, your strength might actually work against you.

"Trying to put all your might into casting a fly is like trying to throw a feather as hard as you can. Force is not the answer—technique is," says Tom Ackerman, director of the L.L. Bean Fly-Fishing School in Freeport, Maine. So we pooled the advice of expert anglers and got their take on the best ways to be a powerful fisherman.

Watch the clock. When you're casting, use the tick-and-tock method to learn how to cast. Imagine you're standing next to a giant clock.

"Keep your elbow at your side and make a fist with your thumb sticking out of the top," explains John Blair, a fly-fishing instructor in Fairfax, Virginia, who devised the tick-and-tock method. Point your thumb at nine o'clock on the imaginary clock—which is straight in front of you. "Now, lift your elbow up and bring your arm back to one o'clock. Say 'tick' as you do this," says Blair. Once your thumb is at one o'clock, say the word "and"—that gives your line time to come back behind you. Finally, say "tock" and briskly bring your thumb back to nine o'clock. "Practice that enough, and you'll develop a good, strong cast," says Blair.

Watch your step. Wading around a river full of slippery rocks may give you a workout you never counted on. "It's probably a good idea to do some balance exercises before you go fishing," says Ackerman. Here's the simplest one: Close your eyes and stand on one foot for as long as you can—at least 30 seconds. Then switch feet. Keep increasing the length of the balancing act by 15 or 30 seconds until you can balance yourself for as long as you want.

Spin a yarn. If you live in the city or don't have a backyard to practice your casts, attach a six-foot piece of yarn to the tip of your rod. "One foot of yarn is about equal in weight to four or five feet of fly line," says Ackerman. Now you can practice your casts in close quarters—and the next yarn you spin will be about the one that got away.

Packing for Your Health

You never know what dangers you're going to encounter in the back-country. "Injuries can occur even with the most stringent preparation," says Dr. Crouse. So instead of packing troubles in your old kit bag, pack a few of these survival essentials.

First-aid kit: You can purchase basic first-aid kits at most camping stores or pharmacies. Or you can put one of your own together. Just make sure it contains adhesive strips, gauze pads, medical adhesive tape, scissors, tweezers, aspirin or another painkiller, moleskin or other foot-care products and iodine water treatment tablets. And don't forget to pack any personal prescriptions you might need.

Skin screens: In the summer, skin burns. In the winter, lips chap. "Be sure to bring along plenty of lip balm," says Dr. Crouse. "And always pack sunscreen: Even on cloudy days, you could be exposing yourself to too much of the sun's rays." And that exposure could lead to painful sunburn or, worse, possibly the start of skin cancer.

Water: "Again, it's a very commonsense thing, but quite a few hikers forget to bring plenty of fresh water and often don't find enough where they're going," Dr. Crouse says. Always bring along at least a couple of water bottles per person if you're going on a day hike. For longer trips consider buying a water purifier, which will leech harmful bacteria out of stream water. But be prepared to spend $60 to $100 for one.

While you're on the trail, remember to drink often—at least every 20 or 30 minutes. "Drink before you feel thirsty. Because by the time you feel thirst, you're already a little dehydrated," explains Dr. Crouse.

wouldn't play football without a helmet, don't do any hiking without proper gear.

Lillard says hikers should seek expert advice from a reputable sporting goods store or wilderness outfitter on what equipment they need for their planned outings. Among the items they should consider are a strong pack (you'll need to learn to adjust it to fit your frame) and an assortment of clothing. Pack waterproof shells for warmth and dryness in wet weather, apparel made from synthetics that wick away moisture from your body, and headgear to keep the sun or rain off or keep your body heat in. And be sure to wear sturdy, comfortable boots that stand ready to support your feet and ankles against the rockiest trails.

Golf

Making Power Par for the Course

Golf looks easy. Think of Chevy Chase as the whacked-out, Zen-master golf pro in the 1980 comedy hit *Caddyshack*. Blindfolded, he hits a perfect chip shot over a water hazard, leaving himself a gimme putt. "Be the ball," Chase cryptically advises his awestruck caddy.

But things aren't always as they seem. After all, Chevy Chase actually seemed funny back then. And as most weekend duffers painfully discover, golf isn't as easy as it looks—especially on your body. After 18 holes of golf, you may indeed feel at one with the ball, but not in any mystical sense. Without proper conditioning and stretching, you can end up feeling like you've spent the afternoon being bashed with a club and bounced off trees.

"Golf doesn't cause injuries. Deconditioned athletes do," says Randy Myers, fitness director at the PGA National Resort and Spa in Palm Beach Gardens, Florida.

Fore Play

Scientific studies of amateur golfers confirm what golf pros will tell you: Most golf-related injuries occur in the back, shoulder, elbow and wrist. And touring pros who stake their career on how strong they play the back nine are not immune from back pain. In one recent year, 59 percent of the injuries reported on the PGA tour were to the trunk—the back and abdominal muscles.

Myers, who has developed conditioning regimens for PGA stars

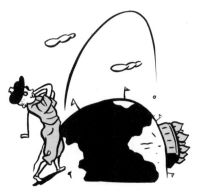

including Gary Player, Corey Pavin and Hale Irwin, says that about half of all golfers eventually suffer an injury. Most can be traced to lack of strength and flexibility in the main muscles used in golf.

Many people mistakenly believe that golf power flows from the shoulders and arms. "For good golfers, 80 percent of their power comes from the legs," Myers says. "For bad golfers, 20 percent comes from the legs."

Pro golfers learn to make the club an extension of their arms. Real golfing power starts in the quadriceps and is translated up through the glutes into the back and stomach muscles. In addition to the key role the legs play in the golf swing, building a strong base is essential given the hurry-up-and-wait nature of the game.

"The best estimates are that you're only playing about 22 minutes of golf during a four-hour round," Myers says. "If you're on your feet for four hours, but you're only playing 22 minutes, the legs really play an important role."

Most golfers want to spend their free time on the links, not in the gym. But hitting the weights once or twice a week will help you play longer and better. If time is tight, Myers recommends doing the following circuit at least once a week. All you need are dumbbells, a bench and a wall. Do two to three sets of 10 to 12 repetitions for each exercise. Get the most out of your rest time between sets by mixing in stretches, abdominal exercises such as crunches, and incline push-ups and dips. (Incline push-ups are the same as regular push-ups except you rest your hands up on a bench instead of on the floor.)

Work the legs first. The key role your legs play on the golf course should be reflected in the gym. Myers recommends incorporating squats and lunges into your regular routine to build strong quads and glutes.

Hit the wall. Start with a five-pound dumbbell in each

hand, and lean against a wall with your back and head flat against it. Bend at the knees so you're in a semi-squatting position. If it feels familiar, it should. "It's basically an upright golf stance," Myers says.

Staying in that position, do standard side raises and front raises. To ensure full range of motion in the rotator cuff, add a variation of an upright row that Myers calls the raised press. Bring the dumbbells straight up to your chin as you would in an upright row. But instead of lowering them, extend your arms straight out in front of you at shoulder level. Then, keeping your arms straight, lower the dumbbells to the starting position. The full motion basically forms a triangle.

Lay down on the job. Next, do a chest fly, which is a variation of the standard bench press. Laying flat on the bench, raise the dumbbells straight up over your body as you would in a bench press. At the top of the motion, rotate your palms inward and bring your hands together over your chest. Rotate them back out, lower and repeat. Finish up with the overhead extension and the triceps extension.

Get in the Swing

Having strong muscles isn't enough to keep you from suffering back pain. You also need to stretch.

To make it easier, Myers has devised a series of stretches that can be done with your golf cart while you wait on the course. The following stretches can help you avoid stiffness, while adding accuracy and power to your shots, says Myers.

Lower-back stretch. Stand facing the side of the cart, about a foot away. Making sure your knees are slightly bent, reach out and grab the handle on the side of the cart. Keeping your

---

Power ⬆ Tip

If your job keeps you on the road, far from your basement gym or local health club, you can still maintain upper-body strength for your golf game.

"You heard it here first: The best upper-body conditioning exercise for golf, bar none, is an incline push-up," says Randy Myers, fitness director at the PGA National Resort and Spa. "I'll tell you why: It strengthens the upper chest, the mid-back, keeps you in a good postural position and also gets extension for the triceps and forearms." If you can't find an exercise bench, use the bathtub or a sturdy desk in your hotel room.

---

arms fully extended, sit back so your buttocks and hips extend out away from the cart. You should feel a stretch in the lower part of your back. Hold for ten seconds. Return to the starting position and repeat two times.

Front-shoulder stretch. Stand at the side of the cart, with your back to the vehicle. With your left arm at shoulder height, reach back and grab the roof post. Holding on to the post, slowly rotate your hips and torso to the right until you feel a stretch in the left shoulder. Hold for ten seconds. Return to the starting position, release your left hand and reach back with your right, grabbing the opposite post of the cart. Holding on with your right hand, turn your torso to the left. Repeat both stretches twice.

Rear-shoulder stretch. Stand about a foot away from the passenger side of the cart, facing the cart. Reach your right hand out and grab the roof post at shoulder height. Slowly rotate your hips and torso to the right, looking over your right shoulder until you feel a stretch in the shoulder muscles. Hold for ten seconds and slowly release. Now move to the other side of the cart and perform the exercise with your left hand. Repeat both stretches twice.

Tennis

How to Court Power

Year-round, whether there are mounds of snow outside or blistering sun, you can flick on the TV and find a good tennis match to watch. Unlike baseball, football, basketball and most other sports, tennis has no prescribed season.

Oh, if you live in Chicago and you only play recreationally on outdoor courts, identifying your seasonal pattern is not much of a problem. But if you live in a climate that's friendly year-round, or if you get lots of indoor play, or if you're a competitive player facing wall-to-wall tournaments throughout the year, you need to artificially enforce an in-season and off-season, says Paul Roetert, Ph.D., administrator of sport science for the United States Tennis Association.

This cyclical change in training emphasis, called periodization, makes for better long-term physical development. While the training cycle for recreational players might follow a yearly pattern peaking in summer, top athletes can fit in four complete cycles a year, peaking for the most important tournaments.

Here's how Dr. Roetert breaks down the phases of tennis training.

• Preparation phase: A minimum of four weeks. Besides your tennis workout, develop a strong aerobic base, emphasizing muscular, cardiovascular and respiratory fitness. Work on your aerobic fitness with jogging or, if you need to go easy on your joints, swimming and cycling. Train heavily in the specifics of tennis.

• Pre-competition phase: A minimum of four weeks. Continue some of the aerobic training, but start emphasizing power with strength training and sprints.

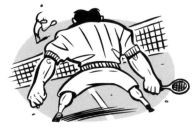

• Competition phase: Three weeks, maximum. Focus on maintaining your strength and endurance. Train heavily in the specifics of tennis. Training load can ease up some if you're playing lots of competitive matches.

• Active rest phase: One to four weeks. First, take a rest from tennis, but keep your fitness up by playing other sports. Then start playing tennis again, with an emphasis on any technique changes you need to make.

Off Court: Your Advantage

Tennis requires a blend of strength, speed and aerobic fitness: Strength and speed, for those rocketlike serves, killer ground strokes and lightning dashes across the court. Endurance, to power yourself through those marathon points—even in the last set of your match. So you need total-body training.

Strength training should involve both the upper and lower body, in particular the shoulders, back, arms, legs and hips. According to Dr. Roetert, the following is an effective exercise sequence for machines and free weights: lat pull-downs, bench presses, upright rows, upper-back flies (these are the same as the bent-over lateral raises described in part two of this book, except they are done on a bench instead of standing), lunges (with or without weights), squats, ab crunches and lying hyperextensions. To do an upper-back fly, lie face down on a bench, chin off the edge, arms hanging straight down from the sides of the bench; holding a dumbbell in each hand with your palms facing each other, slowly lift your arms straight out to the sides as high as you can, then slowly lower them. Dr. Roetert cautions that in the squat, your knees should stay behind your toes and your upper thighs should be parallel to the floor. To do the lying hyperextensions, lie on your stomach, with your arms extended overhead, palms on the floor. If you can, raise your arms and legs at the same time. If that is too difficult, raise your right arm and left leg, then repeat on the opposite side.

Players must warm up and stretch before every workout, says Dr. Roetert. The warm-up can be anything from jogging in place to riding a bike to the gym. After breaking a sweat, stretch all major muscle groups, holding each stretch for a minimum of 20 seconds.

During the actual workout you should complete two sets of 15 repetitions per exercise, resting only 30 seconds between each set. If you are new to strength training, for the first two weeks use weights that allow for completion of 15 repetitions with only moderate effort and give yourself up to 1½ minutes between sets. After this introductory period you should increase the weight until you are barely able to complete 15 repetitions (in good form) in each set.

Strengthening your shoulders and back will help you avoid some of the most common tennis injuries. "I'd say shoulders and backs are numbers one and two," Dr. Roetert says. Strengthening the muscles around the smaller joints—knees, ankles and elbows—also is important.

On Court: Practice Is Perfect

Here are some on-court techniques and drills that will increase your strength, stamina and agility in a tennis-specific way.

Get hopping. This exercise helps you stabilize the body during quick changes of direction, says Dr. Roetert. Tape a hexagon— that's a six-sided figure—to the court, 24 inches on a side. Time yourself: Start by standing in the middle. Jump with both feet over one side of the hexagon and then jump back to the middle. Then do the same for the next side of

> ## Power ⬆ Tip
>
> **Michael Chang, one of the top-ranked tennis players in the world, likes his workouts with a twist.**
>
> **To exercise his obliques (the muscles that run down the sides of the stomach and turn the torso), Chang plays catch with a trainer using a 15-pound medicine ball and rotating just his upper body.**
>
> **"All shots require twisting," says Chang, "so I do more abdominal work than anything else."**

the figure. Continue until you have gone completely around three times. Through the whole exercise you must face in the same direction— you'd never turn away from the net during play, would you?

Dash 20 yards. Dr. Roetert suggests that you time yourself running alongside the court from the baseline to the service line on the opposite side—a distance of exactly 20 yards. This is the farthest you will ever have to run in one burst during a tennis match. Work on accelerating as fast as possible and maintaining your maximum speed.

Curl your bag. Everybody carries a tennis bag. While you're waiting for your partner to show up at the courts, grasp your bag by the handles and use it to simulate dumbbell lifts to strengthen your wrists, upper arms and shoulders, says Dennis Van der Meer, founder and president of the Van der Meer Tennis University on Hilton Head Island, South Carolina, and president of the United States Professional Tennis Registry.

Pick up strength. Many tennis players have learned clever ways to pick tennis balls up off the court with their racquets. Well, notes Van der Meer, why not give your quads a workout between points? Squat to pick up balls with your hands. Or simulate a groin stretch: one knee bent, the other leg straight.

Bowling

How to Have Power to Spare

There's a reason the Great Wallendas don't lug bowling balls around on the high wire. One of those 16-pounders will play hell with your center of gravity. Just imagine what happens when you swing one around in the air regularly.

"The sport of bowling is one of the hardest on your body," says Justin Hromek, a three-time titlist on the professional bowling circuit. "There are very few sports that exert that much pressure on your shoulder, elbow, wrist and back. You're swinging this 16-pound ball, and you have all this weight on one side of your body and nothing on the other side of your body. So it puts a lot of strain on your back and shoulder."

Hromek uses strength training to build muscular endurance and steel himself against injury. He lifts light weights four or five times a week, on days when he's not bowling. He uses a simple barbell set that's easy to deal with on the road.

"I have just a very basic workout," he says. "I do curls, and then I'll do a behind-the-neck press and sometimes a row. For the legs, I use that same curl bar and I do squats. I do them slowly, and I don't go down past 90 degrees—sitting position."

Lifting Your Game

Bowling isn't a cardiovascular activity, but even recreational players can burn 450 calories an hour while they work out the 130 muscles involved. It's a sport people are likely to stick with, too, because it's fun and offers lots of socializing. That may be why one in three Americans plays the sport at least once a year.

But to truly enjoy yourself, you need muscles that are up to the task. The most common maladies among bowlers, doctors say, are tendon and muscle problems in the elbows, forearms, wrists and fingers. For relief, they recommend cross-training as well as strength and flexibility training.

"Bowling's a combination of strength and flexibility," says Carmen Salvino, a 17-time Professional Bowlers Association national champion who's now in his sixties. "You have to have strength and you have to have endurance, because you're out there in the finals for four solid hours twice a day. You might have to walk across 50 or 60 lanes, and you have to carry your bowling balls with you. If you're going to carry four bowling balls across 50 lanes, you'd better be strong."

To meet that need, Salvino favors strength training with low weights and high repetitions to build muscular endurance. "I never went over 100 pounds when I put it on my shoulders, and never went over 25 pounds when I did anything with my arms," says the six-foot-two, 193-pound hall-of-famer.

Bowler Jeff Lizzi, 1992 winner of the Brunswick Memorial World Open, concurs. "I do like a full-body workout—chest, arms, legs, back and stomach," says Lizzi. "When you're in a tournament bowling around 200 games a week, you have to throw the first shot as good as the last shot. It's most important to have your arms strong. And a lot of bowling is in the lower body, giving you the leverage to throw the ball.

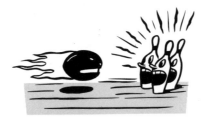

"I do a lot of bench presses, arm curls and flies, triceps pull-downs or extensions. I do leg extensions, leg curls and a lot of lunges—those help a lot, because they also stretch the muscle out."

Like Salvino, he does his weight lifting with low weights

and high repetitions. He also gets aerobic exercise on treadmills and stair-climbing machines.

Better Safe Than Sore

Bowling, if you're doing it right, is not a contact sport. And while bowling is considered a low-risk activity, it's still possible to get hurt. Lewis A. Yocum, M.D., a sports medicine specialist at the Kerlan-Jobe Orthopaedic Clinic in Inglewood, California, suggests the following safety reminders.

- Warm up before you play, and do stretches—particularly for the shoulders and back.
- To avoid shoulder strain, keep your backswing under control. Don't let it rise above your head.
- Pick a ball with a comfortable weight. Beginners should start with a lightweight ball. If you feel pain in the shoulder or arm, it might be because your ball is too heavy.
- To prevent blisters and cuts, be sure the finger holes fit comfortably.
- Lift the ball with both hands.
- Wear loose clothing, and make sure your shoes aren't wet and won't stick to the floor. Bowlers need to be able to slide on that last step before the release, and sticking shoes could hurt your knees or back.

Here are more training secrets for a better and safer bowling game.

Strike a balance. Unless you're ambidextrous, bowling—like other one-sided sports—will develop one side of your body more than the other. You can compensate for that during your daily activities.

"If you want great balance, you need to be symmetrical," Salvino says. "If you're developing one side of the body bowling or doing any other sport, then you have to develop the

other side so that the center of gravity stays in the center. I'm right-handed, so I do everything in life left-handed. If I carry a suitcase, I use the left arm. If I open a door, I do it left-handed. When I work out after bowling, I work out left-handed."

Loosen your grip. To protect your wrists, find a comfortable and relaxed grip on the ball, Lizzi suggests. "Throwing a 16-pound ball is a lot of wear and tear," he says. "A bad grip makes you squeeze the ball more, so you put a lot of stress on your tendons and ligaments just to hold onto it. Then you have to *throw* it. So if you get the most comfortable grip, you're less likely to pull tendons or ligaments."

Keep it simple. Salvino favors stretch-cord exercises because the equipment travels so easily. "When I go on the road, I can take these strong hoses in my suitcase, and I don't have to worry about going to a gymnasium—I take it with me," he says. "I work with my legs on them, I work with my arms, pulling side to side, forward to back."

Swimming

Stoke Your Stroke with Strength

No wonder they say, "Different strokes for different folks." Swimming is a wide, wet world of physical conditioning. Swimmers' training needs can vary from highly aerobic to highly anaerobic, depending on the events they decide to specialize in. A 50-meter race, for instance, requires primarily explosive power and strength, while a 1,500-meter competition is mainly endurance-oriented.

All swimmers draw on some combination of strength and endurance, and strength training of some variety is crucial to their training. If you haven't decided which type of emphasis you need, take a look at the events you enjoy most and the events you score best in. Newcomers to strength training should first try a total-body strength regimen on free weights or machines for six to eight weeks, and then graduate to a program that focuses on swimming specifics.

Although swimming is often thought of as an endurance sport, "the fact is that 75 percent of the competitive swimming events are 200 meters or less, and they really require explosive effort," says John P. Troup, Ph.D., former director of medicine and sport science for United States Swimming, the national governing body for competitive swimming, located in Colorado Springs, Colorado. "It's true that swimming requires an endurance base, but swimming is really by nature of its events a sprint type of activity. We know there are high correlations between muscle power—the size of your muscle fibers and how much power you can generate—and how fast you'll be able to swim."

Swimmers can use stan-

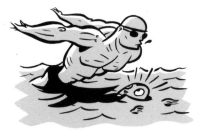

dard free weights, machines, stretch cords and calisthenics in their training, plus swimming-specific equipment like the swim bench, a resistance machine found at some larger YMCAs and fitness and swim clubs that simulates the swimming motion.

Swimming through the Seasons

Certified strength and conditioning specialist John Graham says a swimmer's training is just about a year-round concern. He organizes swimmers' training into three phases designed to reach peak conditioning during the competitive season.

• Off-season: Swimming, plus strength training three times a week, emphasizing muscle development, particularly around the shoulders (which are the most vulnerable to swimming injuries), arms, hips and knees. Lifting starts at 60 percent of repetition maximum and progresses slowly up to about 75 percent.

• Preseason: Time spent swimming increases. Strength training, three times a week, focuses on power and strength gains for competition. Lifting starts at 75 percent and progresses up to 85 percent of repetition maximum. Emphasis should be placed on increased flexibility.

• Competition: Strength training two times a week, at 70 to 85 percent repetition maximum. Daily flexibility training.

Here's a typical lineup of strength-training exercises for swimmers.

Day One—bench presses, incline presses, upright rows, swimmer pull-downs, upper-back flies (these are the same as the bent-over lateral raises described in part two of this book, except they are done on a bench instead of standing), lying overhead triceps extensions, push-ups and an abdominal exercise, such as crunches. To do swimmer pull-downs, stand at a lat pull-down station and use an 8- or 12-inch bar. Start with your arms straight out at shoulder height and lower the bar to your thighs. To do a posterior raise, lie on your stomach on a bench with your chin over the edge and raise dumbbells to shoulder level, straight to the side.

Day Two—squats, leg presses, leg curls, three-way heel raises, dumbbell rows, front lat pull-downs, biceps curls, back extensions and knee lifts. Three-way heel raises are heel raises done with the heels together and toes pointed out, then with feet parallel, then with toes together and heels apart. To do knee lifts, sit on a bench, place your hands behind you for support and extend your legs down toward the floor. Then lift your knees slightly higher than your waistline, with your body forming a V. Lower and repeat.

In the off-season do three sets of 10 to 12 reps. Decrease your reps to 8 to 10 in the preseason and do two to three sets. In-season, keep the reps at 8 to 10 and decrease the sets to two.

Here are more ways to become a more powerful swimmer.

Make like Flipper. A swimmer will typically take a breath every three or four strokes. But as the swimmer gets tired near the end of a race, less of that oxygen gets to his muscles. To improve performance, train your body to endure on less oxygen. An underwater exercise helps: At one side of the pool, take a deep breath, go under and push off. With your arms out front and doing a dolphin kick, try to cross the pool on the one breath. Once you've done it, work on your speed and distance.

Tailor your workout. When you're designing a weight-training program, consider which muscles are important to the strokes you use most. "The legs provide the least amount of propulsion in backstroke and freestyle

Power ⬆ Tip

When you work out on a swim bench, you develop your muscles in precisely the way that swimming demands. But you aren't likely to find such a resistance machine in the standard gymnasium or at the neighborhood pool. For a convenient alternative, jump in the pool with a stretch cord or surgical tubing, suggests Jaci VanHeest, Ph.D., an exercise physiologist for United States Swimming. The cord should be long enough to let you swim 10 to 15 yards from the wall, Dr. VanHeest says.

"A lot of folks in swimming use surgical tubing when they're trying to focus on movement-specific strength or endurance," Dr. VanHeest says. "Typically, you attach it to a belt around your waist, tie the other end of the tube to a starting block and swim part of the way out into the pool. Then you swim against that surgical tubing. You're kind of swimming in place, and you're getting resistance from the tubing."

Sheds a new light on "going nowhere fast," doesn't it?

swimming—only about 20 percent of the forward movement," Dr. Troup says. "But in the breaststroke and butterfly, they become much more important. So leg extensions and curls are recommended."

Pump some rubber. Pick up a set of exercise stretch cords or surgical tubing from a fitness store. Essentially, they're large rubber bands with handles attached that you can use to duplicate free-weight exercises. "You stand and pull against the cord from an anchor point, pulling against the resistance," says Dr. Troup. "The greater the resistance, the more force you have to generate. What you're actually doing is training the recruitment of your muscle fibers in a swiminglike motion."

Skiing

When Power Goes Downhill

As a seasonal sport, skiing can be one of the hardest to stay in shape for. Often as not, we don't allow our bodies any time to prep for a winter of downhill and cross-country fun. But skiing is hard on the body—especially the joints—and experts say to be in shape for it, you should train year-round, not just when the leaves start to turn.

"Year-round training isn't just for world-class skiers anymore," says Robert King, an instructor at the Vail Ski School in Colorado in the winter and a personal trainer who leads a ski-conditioning program at the Vail Athletic Club throughout the year. "If you start to train only a few weeks before the season, you're asking for trouble."

Muscle for Moguls

Luckily, working some ski-specific exercises into your regular fitness routine isn't going to take a lot of effort. Chances are you're already strength-training some of those areas. Here are a few trail markers to get you pointed in the right direction.

Let yourself slide. "Because you're moving laterally when you're skiing, you want to be sure to do a lot of lateral exercises," says King. "Slide aerobics is one of the best ways to go, and some exercise machines work the inner and outer thighs well."

Rely on your quads. Your quads are going to take plenty of punishment when you ski. "And those muscles need to be in good shape, because they help support and protect the

knee. If you don't have good quad strength, you could be inviting knee surgery somewhere down the line," King cautions. So do the exercises that work the glutes, quads, hamstrings and calves—especially squats and lunges, lunges, lunges. "During our training program we do every kind of lunge imaginable—lunges, lateral lunges, reverse lunges, you name it," King says. "It gives you some idea how important quad strength is to skiing."

Be an abdominal snowman. Working the abdominal muscles is just as important as leg work. "Your abs are your foundation," insists Olympic downhill gold medalist Tommy Moe. "A lot of people don't realize how much they use their torso."

King agrees. "In my estimation, the abdominals are equal with the legs as the most important muscle group. So do plenty of abdominal exercises. They are the core of your fitness program."

Improve by leaps and bounds. Bounding exercises simulate skiing movements, and Moe and other skiers make them an important part of a regular ski workout. Try this: Keeping your feet together, hop sideways over a small box (6 to 8 inches high and 12 inches wide)—the action tones the muscles you use for quick turns on skis. Hopping on one leg helps, too, as do tuck jumps—simultaneously jumping straight up and touching both knees to your chest as many times as you can.

Start at the top. As King notes, skiers often neglect muscles above the abs. "But

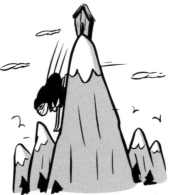

they're all important, too. You need arm, chest and back strength to complement lower-body strength for balance." Good upper-body exercises include push-ups and the bench press, as well as biceps curls and upright rows for arms, shoulders and upper back.

Follow a warming trend. Of course, warming up is an essential part of skiing—but not if it involves an Irish coffee in front of a roaring fire. Before you hit the slopes, do some modified hurdler and hamstring stretches; then take a few runs down a beginner trail. That will get your leg muscles warm, and well it should. Studies have shown that putting cold muscles through rigorous physical activity can reduce their strength by almost 30 percent, on average.

Cross Over

If your brand of skiing is more horizontal than vertical, congratulate yourself on picking one of the best aerobic exercises around.

"You can't beat cross-country skiing," says King. "It's tough, but it's a great workout. When people tell you to cross-train and build more aerobic fitness, one of the first sports they suggest is cross-country skiing, either out on the trail or on a machine that simulates cross-country."

That's great for athletes in other sports. Meanwhile, what are cross-country skiers supposed to do for better cross-training and aerobic fitness? Try these.

Adopt Alpine aerobics. Any form of aerobic exercise will help improve your skiing form. Having a strong heart and powerful lungs will keep you skiing longer and faster.

"The really good aerobic activities for skiing are the ones that continue to work the knees, the upper legs, the lower back," King says.

Mountain biking ranks high on the list, as do running and speed-hiking, which ski champ Moe does. Moe also enjoys kayaking, which helps develop balance and upper-body strength.

Get in-line. If you only do one off-season exercise, make it in-line skating.

"It's probably the number one off-season sport among skiers because it's so great," says

Power ⬆ Tip

When he's in training, Olympic champion Tommy Moe spends hours every day keeping his gold-medal muscles in proper skiing trim. Not surprisingly, the legs are his main focus. "I do a lot of lunges, squats with weights. I also do a ton of jumping exercises." But Moe says the best way to improve your skiing form is to strut your stuff—literally.

"Once I'm finished with most of my leg and ab work, after the box jumps and tuck jumps, I'll spend a good five or ten minutes strutting," Moe says. But he's not talking about the Mick-Jagger-on-stage kind of strut. Moe walks around on his heels with his toes elevated.

The strutting exercise really powers up your ankles and fine-tunes a skier's balance, Moe says. "Plus it strengthens calf muscles. Both are really important if you want to make quick turns on the track—which I do."

King. "The lateral and forward motion of skating, plus the motion that turns the skates, simulates the motions of skiing very well. You really work the muscles in your legs—and even in your feet." When King conducts in-line training, his students attack a variety of terrains. "Don't just skate on flat terrain," he admonishes. "Do a lot of uphill work, work on your maneuverability going downhill—get the most out of it," he says.

Have fun. Whatever form your year-round ski-training routine takes, be sure to vary it. "If it gets boring—or you start to feel like it's something you have to do—I guarantee you won't stick with it," says King. "So make sure your workout isn't all in the club. Mix it up—do indoor work, outdoor sports that use your skiing muscles, do work at home. The more variety you have, the better you'll do."

Basketball

Making Your Power Move to the Hoop

If you wanted to build the perfect basketball player, you could take the explosive speed of sprinter Carl Lewis, the upper-body strength of boxer George Foreman, the vertical leap of high jumper Dwight Stones, the endurance of marathoner Frank Shorter and the soft hands of pro football receiver Jerry Rice.

Or you could just take Michael Jordan.

Few other sports require such a demanding mix of speed, aerobic endurance, physical strength and agility. To play full-court basketball, you have to be in peak condition. And your odds of playing well and remaining injury-free are greatly enhanced if your training program converts the three-point play: resistance training, flexibility and aerobic conditioning.

Lifting Your Game

Hitting the weights can help you hit the boards and hit the open jumper. Just ask Miami Heat center Alonzo Mourning, an NBA all-star who lifts weights two or three times a week. "I'm obsessed with weight training. When you know how much good lifting is doing for your body, it's easy to make a habit of it."

No matter how much weight you lift, odds are you still aren't going to be able to throw down monstrous, rim-rattling dunks like Mourning. But with a little work, you can elevate your game.

Grabbing rebounds

and—for those more vertically gifted—dunking the ball demand explosive leg strength. Chip Sigmon, who worked with Mourning as strength and conditioning coach when Mourning played for the Charlotte Hornets, says building powerful legs is the key.

"The player who has the best vertical jump is the one who can produce the most velocity, the most speed," Sigmon says. "To create velocity, it's just like a jet airplane. It has to have some absolute strength behind it. That absolute strength comes from the jet engine. It's the same in basketball. Where does that speed come from? Well, it comes from the legs."

To increase your vertical jump, you need to build strength, and then speed, in your legs. So start with squats or leg presses, working with heavy weights—about 85 percent of the most you can lift one time, recommends Sigmon. Do 6 to 12 reps and three to four sets.

Once you've built strength through a regular weight-lifting program, add speed. You do that by cutting the weight in half, bringing it down slowly and then exploding through the lifting motion as fast as you can. Sigmon suggests lifting for strength one day and for speed on your second day, or perhaps capping off your regular sets with a speed set.

To build upper-body strength, Sigmon recommends bench presses, incline bench presses, military presses and upright rows. To support your lower back, which takes a pounding in basketball, make sure you do abdominal exercises as part of your regular routine. Orlando Magic center Shaquille O'Neal does 20 minutes of ab work three or four days a week.

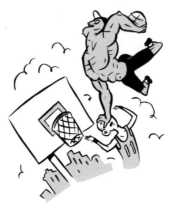

Stretching Your Wings

It wouldn't be stretching the point to call Shaquille O'Neal one of the most feared and dominating players in the NBA. And stretching is one of the things that keeps him that way. "I stretch at least 20 minutes every day, no exceptions," O'Neal says.

That's all-star advice, says Paul M. Steingard, D.O., team physician emeritus with the NBA's Phoenix Suns and adjunct professor with the Department of Exercise Science and Physical Education at Arizona State University in Tempe. "Stretch every day at home," Dr. Steingard says. "That's easy. You don't have to go to a gym to do your stretching. You don't just stretch before a game. Stretching is a year-round thing."

O'Neal works on his legs, back and shoulders—the three main areas stressed by basketball. For recreational ballplayers, Dr. Steingard advises concentrating especially on the quadriceps and hamstrings. Most of the injuries he sees in his private practice in Phoenix are sprained ankles and pulled muscles—especially the quads and hamstrings. Many can be traced directly to lack of flexibility, Dr. Steingard says.

Power ⬆ Tip

Kareem Abdul-Jabbar played in more games—1,560—and scored more points—38,387—than any other player in NBA history. The Hall of Fame center attributes much of his amazing longevity and productivity to flexibility gained through years of studying yoga. But one simple strength-training exercise played a key role in his success, Jabbar says.

"It wasn't weight training, although that was important," the former Los Angles Lakers and Milwaukee Bucks star says. "It was skipping rope."

Jabbar calls jumping rope the perfect exercise for basketball players. "It improves your timing, your vertical jump and your explosive power," he says. "They're all tested and improved by jumping rope. I used a weighted jump rope—that's very good for your explosive power. It helps in your jumping and when you're starting to sprint. It's very good for basketball players of any level."

Running the Fast Break

You need an aerobic conditioning base if you want to play basketball. There's no getting around it. For general fitness, Sigmon advocates 20 to 30 minutes of aerobic exercise, such as running, cycling or swimming, three days a week.

But that isn't enough if you want to be able to run the fast break. "Finish off the workout with a series of 10 to 20 40-yard sprints," Sigmon says. "Because that is the sport of basketball—a series of short sprints. They don't have to be all-out. They can be three-quarters speed. Very seldom in

basketball are you running all-out. It's a controlled sprint."

And although it sounds obvious, if you want to play basketball, you need to play basketball more than once a week, but not daily.

Dr. Steingard advocates playing every other day so that the body has more recovery time. "I'd rather you played more frequently than just every Sunday. That's when you're liable to get in trouble," he says.

It's also a good idea to play "with people of relatively your own ability," Dr. Steingard says. "If somebody says he was the last player cut by the Knicks, don't play with him. Because that's the guy who's going to really try to hurt you."

Softball

How to Be a Power Hitter

Playing softball is a lot like dating. For all the fancy techniques we use for hitting on—or scoring with—our target, nothing improves the odds of getting to first base like a good body.

However, unlike dating, a year-round sport for which single men are *always* in training, softball is seasonal and casual, and few men this side of a major league contract spend enough time preparing for their summer softball careers.

"It's considered such a recreational sport, and that's part of the problem," says Cecil Whitehead, 1990 National Softball Player of the Year, now athletic director for the city recreation department in Valdosta, Georgia. "Guys spend the winter indoors, and then when the company softball team starts up, they run out there without any preparation whatsoever—and fall flat on their faces."

Pulled muscles, torn knees, bad shoulders and sprained wrists and ankles are just a few of the items you'll see in the catalog of woes that belongs to every player who didn't take a few minutes at the gym to prep for his favorite pastime.

Training for the On-Deck Circle

Plain and simple, the difference between being one of the boys of summer and one of the boys on the bench is a preseason workout. Exercise experts say a full-body workout is the perfect complement to any sport. Meanwhile, it's not entirely off-base to spend some extra time working and

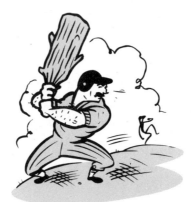

strengthening the specific muscles you need to play ball. Here are a few tips to keep you hard during softball.

Step up to the plates. Time was, ball players were discouraged from doing any weight training, says Whitehead. "It used to be taboo to lift anything—coaches believed all that muscle training would wear you out and ruin your skills," he says. In baseball, timing your swing to a fast pitch will get you a good long hit. But in slow-pitch softball, veterans say muscle is the only thing that will send that ball over the fence.

"I do five days a week with heavy weights—and I mix it up with free and machine," Whitehead says. "Just basic weight training will make a huge difference in your game."

Don't throw the game. When you do your weight training, spend some extra time on your arms and shoulders, advises Dennis Wilson, Ed.D., head of the Department of Health and Human Performance at Auburn University in Auburn, Alabama. They get a lot of punishment when you have to sidearm the ball to first base, or bridge the gap from the right-field fence to your cut-off man.

"It's the nature of the game, unfortunately, that a major area of injury is the throwing muscles," says Dr. Wilson. He says biceps and triceps curls are good all-around arm builders. Also excellent for softball are side lateral raises.

Get your shoulders into the pitch. For batting, pitching or fielding, shoulders also bear a significant brunt from playing ball.

"The muscles that make up the rotator cuff can be easily hurt from swinging and throwing," says Dr. Wilson. So do exercises that work both the shoulders—the aptly named shoulder shrugs, for example—and the rotators.

Dr. Wilson also suggests the "empty can" exercise, a variation on the lateral lift. Instead of lifting the dumbbell straight out from your side, slowly turn your hands so your palms are facing backwards—just as if you were emptying the dregs of your soda can.

Don't perfect your fastball. Although you need speed when you're throwing on the field, be wary of Nolan Ryanesque pitches during practice.

"Speed will come with strength. So when you practice, build the muscles more by throwing long, slow lobs," says Dr. Wilson. And of course, the more you throw, the stronger your arm will be.

Throw spitballs. Some trainers suggest using a weighted softball during training. "You could soak an old softball in water and then do your long, slow throwing exercises," says Dr. Wilson.

Watch your wrists. Fielding and batting power is all in the wrists. Strong wrists and forearms keep a glove steady in the field, and they're paramount at the plate—a strong snap of the wrists can make the difference between a good poke to center field and a grand slam, says softball champ Whitehead.

To target the wrists, Whitehead suggests spending 10 or 15 minutes doing—what else?—wrist rolls, where you hold a dowel with a weight suspended from it. "The weight's on a chain and you slowly twist with your wrists and haul the weight up to the dowel. It's a tough exercise, but it surely does pay off," he says.

Be a home runner. Your legs are the base of any athletic play. In softball, leg strength is essential for a good batting stance, digging out a pop fly or stretching a double into a triple.

"Leg exercises do more than build muscle strength, though," Dr. Wilson says. "They also help protect the legs. Playing softball

---

Power ⬆ Tip

Muscles may be essential for throwing the lumber around, but knowing a few training tricks can put you ahead of the stars on the company softball team. We polled national softball experts for their best advice.

Don't let things slide. 1990 National Softball Player of the Year Cecil Whitehead says recreational players slide too late and end up injuring body parts on bases attached to posts sunk into the ground. First, slide at least a body-length in front of the bag. As you slide, tuck one leg under the other and keep your hands high so you don't jam your fingers. Finally, forget all those pictures of Pete Rose belly-flopping into the bag. Sliding headfirst is too much of a gamble. Always slide feetfirst.

Draw a line in the sand. Hitting the ball perfectly requires good judgment and timing in slow-pitch softball. Softball batting champ Dirk Androff draws a line in the dirt a few feet in front of home plate—a reminder, he says, to hit the ball out front, not once it's over the plate.

Practice with pals. Batting practice is always a must, but skip the batting cages—get a friend to pitch to you instead. As softball Hall of Famer Bruce Meade points out, at a batting cage you're paying for every pitch, so you're more likely to swing at everything, not just what comes over the plate. On the other hand, friends don't let friends ruin their batting eye.

---

is like being a firefighter—you can go from a dead stop to furious activity in a split second. All that stopping and starting takes a toll."

To minimize that toll, strengthen the hamstrings and quadriceps with leg extensions, leg curls, squats and lunges. To build explosive strength, Dr. Wilson suggests sprints or a jump-rope workout.

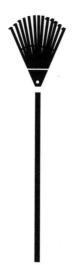

Part Four

Real-Life Power

Improving Sex

Building a Better Bedroom Body

Forget working on that hook shot, and never mind perfecting your parallel skiing. If there's one physical activity men want to be good at—no, be *perfect* at, it's the sport of love.

Like many other vigorous activities, sex requires physical grace and skill if you want to reach your objective. And yes, it does require a certain degree of fitness if you want to be really good.

"The evidence is pretty conclusive. Besides the fact that exercising increases your well-being and confidence—both of which figure into the sexual equation—a regular fitness routine also enhances your physical ability to have sex," says James White, Ph.D., professor emeritus of exercise physiology at the University of California, San Diego.

Science backs that up. In one study of sexual behavior, Dr. White found that men who worked out regularly enjoyed a 30 percent boost in their sexual appetite. But more importantly, the exercisers also reported a significant increase in sexual performance—specifically, they were lasting longer and having more orgasms.

And you thought exercising would only make your muscles hard.

Stretch for Sex

A scene from life: You're sitting in front of the TV, channel-surfing for the game, when your remote accidentally lands you on a free preview of the sex channel. Suddenly, you've forgotten all about the game. Right now, you just want

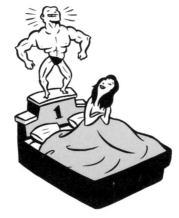

to know how those incredibly skilled actors managed to get into that position.

But you'll never know, because just then your significant other marches in, wondering what all the moaning's about. You switch channels so fast you get a cramp in your thumb. A bit sullen now, you watch the game, but you're still wondering: How'd they do that?

The answer is flexibility, chum.

"If you want to do well—and keep from hurting yourself—in any physical endeavor, you have to have flexible, supple muscles. It doesn't matter whether it's basketball or sex," says Jeff Friday, a strength and conditioning coach at Northwestern University in Evanston, Illinois. So, unless you want to end up with, say, a groin pull in the midst of an Olympic love-making session, take a few minutes every day to limber up those libidinous muscles.

Eric Gronbech, Ph.D., professor of physical education at Chicago State University who researches the link between fitness and libido, recommends trying the following stretches to get you started. If you have a fairly new mattress, it's perfectly okay to do these stretches on the bed. But if your mattress has a furrow in it from years of, ahem, overuse, do these stretches on the floor. And then go out and buy a new mattress.

Raise some calves. Men have a tendency to overflex their calves in the heat of passion, resulting in muscle spasms a bit lower in your body than you might have been expecting, says Dr. Gronbech. You can corral potential calf problems by lying flat on your back on the bed, with one leg bent, foot flat against the mattress. Keeping the opposite leg straight, raise it as far as you can, until it's pointing toward the ceiling. Now flex your foot, pointing it toward your chest. Hold the stretch for a ten-count, relax, then do it two more times. Now switch legs.

Arm yourself. Certain positions—the missionary leaps to mind—put quite a bit of stress on your shoulders, says Dr. Gronbech.

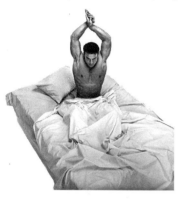

So do a shoulder flexor: Sit up, cross your wrists, then raise your arms above your head as though you were about to be tied to the headboard (hmm, *there's* an idea). Now, straighten your arms and extend them back behind your head as far as you can, while still keeping your wrists crossed. Hold the stretch for a count of ten, relax, and repeat two more times.

Float like a butterfly. No two ways about it—your groin muscles work overtime in the sack. The best way to keep them flexible and avoid embarrassing and untimely muscle cramps is with a butterfly stretch. Lie flat on

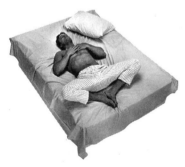

your back in bed, knees bent, feet flat on the mattress. Pull your heels toward your buttocks; now turn your ankles so the soles and heels of your feet are touching one another. Your knees should naturally point out to the sides. Now let gravity do its thing—let your knees slowly drop toward the bed. When they're as far apart as possible, hold for a count of ten, then bring your knees back up. Relax, repeat twice.

Be hip in bed. What do an F-14 and your sex life have in common? Neither one gets anywhere without thrust. The F-14 relies on a jet engine, your libido depends on the thrust

generated by your hips. To get hip to great sex, try this: Stretch your legs out straight, spread them apart, then lean forward from the hips as far as you comfortably can. Keep your legs relaxed and

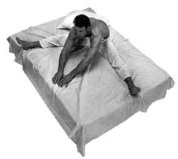

your feet upright. For stability, keep your hands in front of you. Hold for a count of ten, relax, and repeat twice.

The Great Sex Workout

Having a well-muscled body can improve your sexual performance in two ways. First, being in good shape will allow you to last longer. Second, the better you look, the more likely you are to attract partners interested in lasting longer with you. Here's all you need to get rock hard, right now . . . and then again, later.

Exercise abs for amore. Along with your hips, your abdominals help power the thrusting motion so useful during sex. A basic crunch will serve you in good stead. Do three sets of 10 and work your way up from there. "If you can get up to three sets of 20 repetitions, you'll have all the thrusting strength you'll need for sex," says Dr. Gronbech.

Be a muscle missionary. Just as the shoulders need to be stretched, they—along with the arms—also need to be strengthened. If you're on top, you need to hold yourself up as long as you stay up. Collapsing onto your partner because your arms gave out is hardly the kind of climax most guys imagine. Push-ups are the most natural choice for sex-training. In the weight room you can build up your shoulders with—what else?—shoulder shrugs, as well as upright rows.

Treasure your chest. In the film *Kiss of Death*, actor Nicolas Cage portrayed a volatile crime boss named Little Junior Brown who bench-pressed strippers to stay fit. While your partner might offer more than a little resistance to that offbeat training idea, doing bench presses the conventional way can certainly help your love life. Although your chest does minimal work under the covers, Dr. Gronbech reminds us that developing a better physical self pays major psychological dividends. "It allows you to have a more traditionally masculine appearance—you'll look better and feel better about yourself," he says. "It's very useful for attracting a sex partner, in a cosmetic sense if nothing else."

Remember: All muscles matter. Finally, just as a good lover never focuses too long on any one part of his partner's anatomy, when you're working out, don't neglect the rest of the muscles in your body. "During sex there might be a few muscles that work harder than others, but from an overall performance standpoint, be sure you're doing a full-body workout—because sex really is a full-body experience," says Dr. Gronbech. And the more you can do with your entire body under the weights, the better you'll do with that body between the sheets.

Amorous Aerobics

They may not rank number one, but your heart and lungs are a close second on the list of organs important for great sex. "When we did our studies, we found a direct correlation between aerobic activity and sexual performance," says Dr. White. And no wonder: Aerobic activity—figure on three to four sessions a week of 30 to 45 minutes each—is the single

Powerful and Plentiful Orgasms

In the arena of sex, there's one muscle group you want to be sure to work—but you'll never find a circuit machine for it. The muscles in question are the pubococcygeus, or PC, muscles. Besides performing such handy tasks as anchoring the base of the penis to the pelvis and stopping the flow of urine on command, the PCs also contract like crazy during orgasm.

Many experts say that by exercising the PC muscles, you can unlock the door to a whole new bedroom of sexual potential—one where you can prevent premature ejaculation, control the timing and intensity of orgasm and even develop the capacity for multiple orgasms.

But before you do any of these things, you need to strengthen those PCs with a series of exercises called Kegels, named after the doctor who first devised them. Alan Brauer, M.D., a psychiatrist, sex therapist and director of the Brauer Medical Center in Palo Alto, California, recommends that for starters, you should do five sets—10 reps per set—of each of the following Kegels. Each week, add 5 reps per set, until you're doing 30 reps per set.

• Slow clenches. Squeeze your PCs exactly as if you're trying to stop the flow of urine. Hold each clench for a slow count of three.

• Flutters. Clench and relax as fast as you can.

• Push-outs. Bear down on your PCs as though you were trying to force out those last few drops of urine. You'll know you're doing it right when you get your lower abdominals into the exercise.

best way to improve cardiovascular fitness and train your heart and lungs so you don't hit the wall in the final moments. Try these.

Work out with your woman. There

Once you've reached your 30 rep-per-set goal, try these advanced exercises.

• **Super Kegels.** Tighten the PCs and hold that clench for a full 20 seconds. Don't give up if you start to feel the clench fading—just keep renewing the contraction. Do ten Super Kegels spread out over the course of a whole day.

• **Towel raises.** This is one PC exercise that wouldn't be very P.C. of you to do in public, since it requires an erection. Once you have one, gently hang a light washcloth over the end of your penis. Now, using the PC muscles, make your penis jump up and down ten times. As your strength increases, add more weight—move up to a hand towel, then a bath towel.

After a few weeks you should experience firmer erections and more pleasurable contractions during orgasm. But more importantly, Kegels give you finer control over your ejaculations. As you reach the point of no return, by clenching your newly strengthened PCs—with one long squeeze or two medium squeezes, just like tapping a brake pedal—you can bring ejaculation to a screeching halt. Then you can take a long, deep breath and continue with the business—or pleasure—at hand.

If you've been training with Kegels and you can hold the squeeze for several seconds, you can achieve orgasm without ejaculation or losing your erection. Admittedly, this takes practice, and the first few times you try it may not yield the most satisfying results. But the more you try it, the better you'll get. More importantly, you'll be working toward that Holy Grail of sexual achievement, multiple orgasms.

may not know: When her face is flushed at the end of the workout, it may not be entirely from exercise. In a study of women, Chicago State University researchers learned that almost one in four had experienced sexual arousal or even orgasm while exercising. Step aerobics, anyone?

Walk for your woman. There's an old adage: "It's all right to get your appetite walking around town, just as long as you eat supper at home." And like most sayings, it contains a kernel of truth.

"Walking is a good, light aerobic exercise, and certainly won't hurt as a libido lifter," says Dr. White. Just make sure it's part of a more involved workout. In Dr. White's study, men who only walked didn't report nearly the sexual increases of men who walked *and* combined it with more vigorous exercises like running, swimming and weight training.

Take the stairway to heaven. When exercise trainers say stair-climbing can build explosive power, they're not exactly referring to sex. Nevertheless, a few sessions on the stair-climber at your club, or running the stairs once or twice a week at the office, will put some spring in your sexual stride. Other good aerobic jump starts include swimming and cycling.

Have more sex. It may not be as aerobically powerful as an hour on the stair-climber, but sex does qualify as an aerobic activity—and the more sex you have, the more you can have. "It's like any activity—the more you do it, the better you get," says Dr. Gronbech. "If your sexual frequency is a few times a week, you're much better off—in a lot of ways, obviously—than the man who only has sex once a month."

are some obvious reasons to work out together. You get to spend more time together, and you're doing something that makes each of you look and feel better. But here's something you

Doing Chores

Getting Ready for Work

If you're like most homeowners, working out on the weekend usually means working out in the yard, on the roof or in the basement, trying to keep your house in order. You may find yourself asking: Who needs a gym?

Boxing great George Foreman, for one. In 1994, when Foreman regained his heavyweight title after 20 years, the middle-age boxer made yard work an integral part of his comeback workout. To help hone his legendary punching power, Foreman spends hours at his Texas ranch working with a pick and shovel.

"I'll measure out five feet square and I'll dig. I'll keep digging until I get that hole maybe four feet, then I'll cover it up and go on to another. Then I'll get a wheelbarrow and push rocks back and forth," Foreman says.

After that, Foreman hits the woodshed, chopping logs with a hatchet. "When people say I'm out there working on the ranch, I'm really training," he says.

Who are we to argue with the champ? Doing chores makes for a strenuous workout—hauling firewood into the mudroom, raking a square mile of leaves, yanking the lawnmower to life. And on top of this, you're supposed to hit the weights three times a week?

Fit for Life

Well, yes. Not even George Foreman relies exclusively on yard work for power in the ring—it's just an addition to a more formal workout. And that formal workout is what gives him the strength to spend all those hours

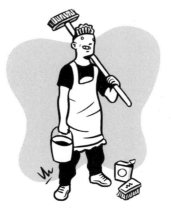

digging and refilling ditches.

"This is one of the reasons why men should be on a regular fitness program—not just to look good and be in shape for their favorite sports, but also to be in shape when it comes time to do some real physical work," says John Amberge, an exercise physiologist at the Sports Training Institute in New York City.

Here are a few exercises designed to help you avoid some of the most common domestic pitfalls.

Twist and shout. Amberge says reverse trunk twists are great for your oblique abdominals—those muscles you use for push-me/pull-me activities like raking leaves or wrestling with the lawn mower.

To do them, lie on your back on the floor, arms straight out to the sides, palms down. Bend your knees, placing your feet flat on the floor. Now, with legs and feet together, slowly lower them to the left until your left thigh touches the floor. Hold for a moment, then raise your legs back to the starting position and switch sides. Do 15 to 20.

Row to mow. Mowing is another great outdoor exercise that burns plenty of calories—assuming you're using a push-mower, of course. But to take advantage of the benefits of being a lawnmower man, you'll need to do more than twists. Spend some time training your upper back muscles, too, using one-arm dumbbell rows, says Chip Harrison, strength and conditioning coach at Pennsylvania State University in State College. You'll know you're working those muscles when you can pull-start your mower in one yank. This exercise also helps when it comes time to rev up the chainsaw in the fall.

Stand with a dumbbell in one hand, and bend at the waist. Place the knee and the hand opposite the one with the dumbbell on a bench or chair for support, keeping your back parallel to the floor. Your other

Scoring Your Chores

So you spent the whole week doing odd jobs around the house, and now you're kicking yourself because you didn't have time to get out and exercise. Don't sweat it. You may well have burned more calories doing chores than engaging in your favorite weekend activity. Check out the chart below and see for yourself.

All numbers below are based on calories burned per hour for a 180-pound male.

Chore	Calories Burned	Activity	Calories Burned
Carpentry	270	Sex	240
Chopping wood	414	Golf	411
Digging (with shovel)	701	Cross-country skiing	666
Gardening (digging, hoeing)	576	Tennis (singles)	522
Mowing lawn	486	Brisk walking (3.5 mph)	432
Painting	378	Bicycling (15 mph)	600
Trimming hedges	378	In-line skating	550
Washing car	270	Volleyball	396

knee should be straight, but not locked. The arm with the dumbbell should hang freely. Raise the dumbbell until it touches the side of your chest. Hold for one count, then lower. Do 8 to 12 reps, then repeat with the other arm.

Be a pick-up artist. For the muscles in the middle back and shoulders—so handy when you're rearranging your crates of stuff in the garage—try upright dumbbell rows, says Amberge.

Flex your hips. When you're hauling junk around, your abdominals and hip flexors carry their share of the load, too. You can exercise them with flat-bench leg lifts.

Sit on the end of a flat exercise bench and grab the sides for support. Put your back flat against the seat of the bench, but raise your neck and shoulders slightly. Now extend your legs parallel to the floor, slightly bend your knees and raise your legs until they form a right angle to your body. Hold for a moment, then slowly lower them until they're at a 45-degree angle, halfway to the bench. Do two sets of 10 to 12 lifts.

Dig your work. George Foreman can tell you: If you want strength, digging can give it to you—in spades. But ounce for ounce, digging is also one of the most exhausting—and potentially injuring—chores you can do. "Besides the strain shoveling can have on the heart, it can also injure the back if you don't do it correctly," says Scott Donkin, D.C., a chiropractor in Lincoln, Nebraska, and author of *Sitting on the Job* and a series of brochures on ways to improve daily physical activities.

So when you take spade in hand, put your dominant hand as far up on the handle as possible. Your other hand should be about 18 inches down from the top of the handle. Push with your legs and arms, not your back or shoulders. Once you have your load of dirt, hold your head up and be sure to pivot your feet when you turn to deposit it—don't twist your back or your knees.

Driving a Hammer Harder

Hitting the Nail on the Head

As far as the average guy is concerned, Peter, Paul and Mary hit it right on the head: If you had a hammer, you *would* swing it in the morning, the evening—heck, you'd probably swing it all over this land, if you didn't have a hundred other things to do.

Men love hammers, and why not? They're a simple, universal sign of power and industry. Taking one in hand, you immediately feel in control of the situation, whether you're about to pitch in at a barn raising or hang a picture frame in your den. You savor the moment as you balance the nail against the wood, draw the hammer back and . . .

BAM!

Hit the wall, leaving an ugly, black dent. Cursing, you draw back and . . .

BAM!

Graze the nail, bending it at a 45-degree angle. Annoyed, you grab a new nail, hold it steady with one hand while drawing the hammer *way* back with the other and . . .

BAM!

Hit the nail dead-on. Only, it's the nail attached to your thumb. And it's slowly turning black. Eyes shut, cheeks flushed, brow sweating, you jam the thumb in your mouth, looking for a moment like Dizzy Gillespie. The moment passes, the pain subsides and you promise yourself once again that you *will* learn how to hit the nail the right way—strong and straight and true.

Unfortunately, if you only handle a hammer once a year, the odds of learning to hit a nail harder are as slim as a finishing nail.

"The single biggest way to get good with a hammer is to use the thing as often as possible," says Jim Little, an organizer with the United Brotherhood of Carpenters and Joiners of America and himself a carpenter of 25 years. "There's a lot of trial and error involved—and a lot of going home with a throbbing thumb, but eventually, you'll get the knack and develop your timing."

Nailing the Technique

You don't have to go out and join the union just to be handy with a hammer. Little says there are a few tricks you can bear in mind the next time you take hammer in hand.

Keep your eye on the nail. Like other activities that involve clubs, hammering is a sport of timing and eye-hand coordination.

"Look at sports like baseball or golf, where you really need to keep your eye on what you want to hit," says Little. "It's the same principle with hitting a nail." But Little stresses that you should really concentrate on the head of that nail. "Your hand basically follows your eye. If you focus strictly on the nail, you'll hit that sweet spot and drive it straight and true," he says. "But if you're worried about your thumb, why sure enough you're gonna glance at your thumb and—bang!—that's where the hammer will go."

Watch your swing. Most men think the higher they bring their hand back, the harder they'll hit the nail. Think again, says Little.

"The further the hammer is away from the nail, the less likely you are to hit that rascal, no matter how hard you swing,"

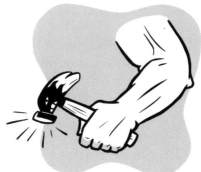

he says. "It's not the swing that counts, it's the contact." As a rule of thumb, don't bring the hammer back more than two feet from the nail. "So what if it takes you two or three strokes to drive the nail? Two or three well-hit strokes are going to get the job done better—and feel a lot more satisfying—than taking a humongous swing," says Little.

Let the handle help. Another way amateur hammerers lose nailing power is by not exploiting the laws of physics.

"When you hold a hammer, I say hold it as close to the bottom as possible. Then when you swing, you're using the full length of the hammer—the arc will be longer and you'll deliver more force to the nail—without having to swing very hard," says Little. Practice this technique first, though—the lower you hold the handle, the more likely it is to slip out of your grasp on the back swing. "Until you get pretty good, make sure there are no windows behind you," jokes Little.

Build muscle. Of course, having some muscle power does help.

"In any activity where you're using a club or a racquet, it's good to do exercises to increase arm and grip strength," says Pennsylvania State University strength and conditioning coach Chip Harrison. To improve grip and forearm strength, you can use spring-loaded grip trainers or squeeze a tennis ball or rubber ball.

For upper-arm strength, try the aptly named hammer curl—a dumbbell exercise in which you hold the dumbbell like a hammer, raise it to your bicep, then slowly lower it. The exercise is similar to the hammering motion. But the extra weight of the dumbbell ensures that you'll have a better hammering strength nailed down in no time.

Tool Time

Being strong with a hammer doesn't depend on physical strength alone—it depends just as much on the type of hammer you're using.

"I don't care if it's been handed down for seven generations or it's the newest tool made out of the latest material—if that hammer doesn't fit your hand, it'll do you no good," says carpenter and union organizer Jim Little. "There are about 75 different kinds of hammers out there—one of them has got to fit you." Here's what to look for next time you hit the hardware store.

• *Heft:* The hammer has to have some weight to it, but not so much that it fatigues you. "Most guys are pretty comfortable with a 16-ounce head, but you have to pick up a lot of different hammers to get the feel of it. If the hammer feels like it's going to drop straight to the floor every time you relax your arm, it's too heavy," says Little.

• *Handle:* Most hammer handles are a little over a foot long and about 1½ inches wide, but Little urges shoppers to try their hand at several hammers. "If you're a big guy, you want a longer-handled hammer. There's one out there with a 22-inch handle and a giant head on it—we call it a warhead. That might be good for a big guy, but average-size guys want to stick with an average-size handle. You should be able to close your fingers around it."

• *Grip:* Most new hammers have a rubber grip on the handles. Little says these are best for amateur carpenters. But if you happen to have a wood-handled hammer, Little passes on this old carpenter's trick. "Take some time with a knife and shave the handle a little bit so that it fits your hand comfortably," he says. "It might take you months to get it right, but then you'll have a hammer custom-made for your hand—and it'll serve you for a lifetime."

Getting a Grip

How to Have a Firm Handshake

As a man, you never know when you're going to have to shake someone's hand, wrestle a lug wrench to change a flat or clamber hand-over-hand across a bamboo bridge spanning a thousand-foot drop into a piranha-filled river.

Okay, maybe that last scenario is more likely for Indiana Jones than for your average Mr. Jones from Indiana. But the fact is, at any given moment in this life, you may have to lend a hand—and when you do, you want it to be strong, firm and full of confidence.

Who among us has not been put off by a limp handshake or impressed by a firm one? When we see a pal or colleague about to lose control of a situation, our first impulse is to scream, "Get a grip!" You spend your life trying to get the upper hand in any situation—or at the very least, to get your affairs well in hand. And when you do, you have the world by the throat—or some other even more vulnerable part of the male anatomy.

Become a Handy Man

Luckily, we live in a hands-on world, so building hand strength is easily within our grasp.

Any weight-lifting exercises that involve pulling movements—chin-ups, lat pull-downs and dumbbell rows, for example—build firm grip strength, says Northwestern University strength and conditioning coach Jeff Friday. "In any weight lifting where you're gripping the bar and pulling the weight, you're exer-

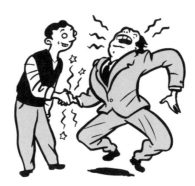

cising those muscles—it can be as simple as that," he says.

Of course, there are other ways to target your grappling muscles exclusively. Here's how.

Grasp for power. Okay, so maybe the secret to a great grip isn't *all* in the hands. When you tighten your grip, feel along your arm. "All those muscles in your forearm are tensing up, adding strength to your grip," says Pennsylvania State University strength and conditioning coach Chip Harrison. You can add strength to them by doing an exercise called a weight-plate finger raise. Try saying that three times fast—more importantly, try *doing* it eight or ten times, slowly.

Hold an Olympic weight plate in each hand by grasping the raised edge of the plate with your four fingers and pressing your thumb against the flat side of the plate. Find a weight that you can handle for ten repetitions. Stand straight, palms inward, arms by your sides.

Straighten your fingers to lower the plate. Now close the fingers, raising the plate as high as you can. As you get stronger, switch from a 10-pound weight to 25 or even 45 pounds.

Put the squeeze on. The best overall grip strengthener is any exercise that gets you flexing your fingers and hands. Spring-loaded grip trainers come in handy, but if you can't find one that fits right, don't despair.

"There are plenty of items around the house you can use," Harrison says. "For instance, squeezing a tennis ball or a rubber ball is a good exercise to improve your grip. You can have one at your desk and use it while you're working."

Develop putty power. If your grip is already too mighty for a mere fuzzy yellow ball, check out your sporting goods store for the newest, most effective—and coolest—hand tools. Take silicone rubber, a pliable putty that offers plenty of strength-training resistance for about ten bucks. Our favorite, Power Putty, even comes in a neat, fist-shaped container and is available for about nine dollars from Brainstorms, a mail-order catalog (call 1-800-621-7500).

Getting a Game Grip

If you can't imagine yourself setting aside time or money to exercise your hands exclusively, the best thing to do is take up an activity that exercises the hands for you—such as politics.

On the other hand, you'll probably enjoy sports and games more. "With the exception of something like soccer, there are very few sports that don't involve good hand strength. Most sports that use an implement to catch or hit a ball will improve your grip strength," Friday says. "Just playing those sports can improve your grip." Here are some of the best examples.

Be a racqueteer. Racquet sports like tennis, squash and racquetball are ideal grip builders. "It's not only a matter of having strength to hold the racquet, but you're also turning the racquet to put spin on the ball—that really works a lot of the forearm muscles," says Harrison.

Play ball! For that matter, any sport that involves a ball and some kind of club is bound to work your hands. "Baseball, softball and golf build hand strength the same way the racquet sports do," Harrison says.

Rock on. If you think *Mountain Climbing* is just a classic rock album, think again. Outdoor sports like rock climbing toughen hands up fast and help strengthen your fingers tremendously. Take this warning in hand, though: "Rock climbing is a hard sport and takes time to be proficient in," says

How to Be a Rubber-Band Man

Even if you've devoted tons of energy to clenching your way to an iron grip, chances are you haven't spent enough time unclenching—working the muscles that allow you to open your hands.

"Men don't really spend a lot of time with specific exercises that involve finger extension, but your hands wouldn't be much good without them," says Pennsylvania State University strength and conditioning coach Chip Harrison.

Luckily, there's a simple, convenient and totally inexpensive way to exercise those muscles.

Got a rubber band?

Find a good thick one—there are probably dozens in your desk drawer. Now make your hand into a "C" shape and wrap the rubber band around the ends of your fingers and thumb—just above your knuckles. If you relax your hand, the rubber band should pinch the hand closed (if it doesn't, find a stronger one or wrap the band around your fingers twice).

Now slowly force your hand open. You'll feel the muscles in your forearms doing their thing. Do about ten repetitions, then switch hands.

Harrison. Besides the fact that you can cut your hands up pretty well, you can also get tendinitis in your fingers if you overdo it. Take your time.

Do the shuffle. For those hard-to-work muscles that make a hand more nimble, pick up a deck of cards. Practicing shuffling or card tricks will vastly improve manual dexterity over time. Just remember that if you decide to practice during a friendly card game with the guys, it could turn into an expensive way to build hand strength—especially if the hand you play is weak.

Powering Up at Work

How to Beat Fatigue Sitting Down

Unless you spend your 9:00 to 5:00 hours, say, fighting oil fires or performing some other intensely physical task, chances are you don't get much of an on-the-job workout. More likely, you sit at your desk for hours on end, performing the same simple tasks over and over, such as checking the clock to see if it's 5:00 yet.

Let's be real: The office is not the most conducive atmosphere to feeling physically powerful. And if the most energetic thing you do all day is dash down the hall for a meeting, or eat your lunch so fast you'd think you were trying to qualify for an Olympic event, then you need to start figuring out ways to stay strong on the job.

Skip On-the-Job Straining

First off, understand that being deskbound can be a detriment to your fitness in ways you probably didn't even know existed.

"Just sitting in one position or doing simple tasks over and over—working the computer, talking on the phone—can cause injuries that will affect your performance elsewhere in life," says Chris Grant, Ph.D., a researcher at the Center for Ergonomics at the University of Michigan in Ann Arbor.

And that's a problem. When the whistle blows, you want to be ready to hit the gym or do your part for the company softball team, not be hunched over in pain, unable to flex a muscle. Here's how to stay invigorated throughout the day—and ensure that the only knot you'll feel at work is the one in your power tie.

Change positions. The single biggest reason office workers get stiff muscles is that they hold one position too long, says Dr. Grant. "You really shouldn't hold one position longer than 10 minutes at a time. After that, you'll start to suffer from static exertion—you'll feel a funny kind of burn or a stiffness in the muscles," she says. If you get to that point, it's too late, so shift your position or take a small break every 10 or 15 minutes.

"If you just give yourself a small rest— even 30 seconds every ten minutes—it can make a difference. Not only are you helping to prevent physical fatigue, you're also throwing off some psychological fatigue as well," Dr. Grant says. So take a break—get up, walk around the building or, better yet, take a stroll outside and get some fresh air. "People who sit all day have a lot of back problems, but people who stand and sit a lot have the healthiest backs," says Dr. Grant. Be one of them.

Create a cockpit. One trick experts recommend is to lay out your work area like the cockpit of an airplane. "You look at a cockpit, and you see that everything is within easy reach—nothing requires you to overextend or try to move in two different directions to accomplish a task," says Dr. Scott Donkin, a chiropractor in Lincoln, Nebraska. "You can lay your work tools on your desk the same way."

Dr. Donkin suggests keeping everything that you use often—phone, computer, stapler—within the sweep of an outstretched hand. "Beyond that circle of use, you'd position

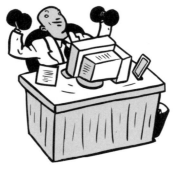

other items that you use less frequently—close by so you can reach them as needed, but not right in your way," he says. Always put items with respect to your dominant hand. If you're right-handed, position the phone on your left side and hold the receiver with your left hand. Your right hand is then free to write or take notes, says Dr. Donkin.

Do a tension check. Mental stress—especially at work—often migrates into your muscles, and you won't know it until you're literally tied up in knots. Every hour at least, see if you have tension somewhere in your body. Pay attention to your hands, shoulders, arms, neck, even your face—when stress hits, we often clench our jaws. If you find tension, take a moment to close your eyes and relax.

Workout for Work

Even if your work space is an ergonomist's dream, you may still occasionally find yourself with a nasty crick in your neck or a stiff arm that won't loosen up. "If it's a busy day and you're stressed out, you can easily end up with strains and pains, despite your best efforts," says Dr. Grant.

To keep you limber, here are a few stretches recommended by Dr. Donkin. Do them as you need them. If you have joint problems or previous physical conditions that stretching might aggravate, talk to your doctor before trying any of these stretches.

Take a micro-break. Assuming you have a chair that reclines slightly (no more than a 45-degree angle)—and won't tip over when it does—Dr. Donkin recommends this tension-relieving break: Lean back in your chair and stretch your arms and legs out. Now wiggle your fingers and toes. Close your eyes, breathe in deeply and slowly and smile. "It's great for relieving muscle tension in your body and improving circulation," Dr. Donkin says.

Get stress off your chest. To relieve tension in your chest and upper back, clasp your hands behind your head, elbows pointing up, and push your palms together. Hold for 30 seconds.

Get your neck stretched. Tilt your

Kicking Bad Work Habits

When you go into work tomorrow, conduct a spot inspection of your work habits. "Some of the simplest motions can cause muscle strain and fatigue—you probably don't even know you're doing them," says the University of Michigan's Dr. Chris Grant. The worst offenders of these worktime bad habits include:

• **Cradling the phone between your ear and shoulder.** "Switch the handset from hand to hand during long phone conversations. Better yet, get a telephone headset," says Dr. Grant.

• **Bending your wrists back when working a keyboard.** "Try to keep your hands and forearms in a straight line," says Dr. Grant.

• **Bending your head back to look at a monitor.** "When you look straight on, the monitor should be no higher than eye level. Many people are more comfortable with the monitor directly on the work surface. If you're constantly tilting your head back to look at it—and people with bifocals do this a lot—don't adjust your head, adjust the monitor," says Dr. Grant. Experiment with raising it or lowering it until you're able to work with your head and shoulders relaxed. Use a copy stand aimed right at your face if you often work from paper.

---

head slowly from one side to the other—don't move it in a circle. Hold each stretch for a count of three. Repeat five to ten times.

Go lower for your back. Sitting in your chair, slowly bend your upper body forward until your head is almost between your knees. Hold for a few seconds, then sit up.

Fight stiffness with your fists. Make a tight fist and hold it for a second. Then spread your fingers as far apart as you can. Hold for five seconds.

Take a deep breath. Finally, devote a few minutes to deep breathing exercises. Breathe in slowly through your nose, hold for two seconds, then exhale through your mouth. Repeat several times or until you feel relaxed.

Lifting Heavy Objects

Getting Back to Basics

It's one of the unwritten rules of being a man. If another guy helped you move—it doesn't matter how many years ago it was or how little stuff you had at the time—you are eternally obligated to help him move. Even if he now has a three-story Victorian house filled with solid oak furniture and—just for fun—a grand piano.

When you were younger, helping buddies move was no big deal. A few hours of lifting, followed by an evening of free pizza and beer. But now, when the phone call comes, you wince, harboring secret, shameful thoughts of violating the sacred rule under the pretense of being out of town for the weekend.

It doesn't have to be that way. With exercise and a little know-how, you can get back in the moving game without worrying about throwing out your back.

Building a Support System

First off, if you're trying to build a stronger back, back up a minute and look at the bigger picture.

"A good back doesn't depend on back muscles alone. There are a lot of other muscles that come into play and help support the back when it's doing any kind of lifting," says Dr. Scott Donkin, a chiropractor in Lincoln, Nebraska. "Since we walk on two legs and not four, there's a need for critical balance against gravity. The back is the

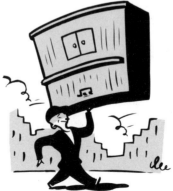

foundation of that balance, but it's not much good without the abdominals, the quads and hamstrings and, of course, the back muscles."

Obviously, those are muscles you should be exercising and strengthening on a regular basis. Here are a few exercises to get you started.

Tune the torso. The real secret to power lifting is not so much in the arms and legs as it is in the torso—specifically, your abdominal and lower back muscles. And for the back, few exercises are as good as the back extension. For your abs make sure crunches are part of your workout—as Dr. Donkin explains, your abdominal muscles lend vital support to the back, especially when you're carrying stuff.

Give your legs some lift. Once you have the package in hand, your quads and hamstrings need to hold up under pressure, says Northwestern University strength and conditioning coach Jeff Friday. To keep them toned, do squats and lunges with a barbell resting across the back of your shoulders.

Get a grip. Arm and hand strength play a pivotal role in lifting, by letting you hold onto the object in question. To strengthen your forearm and grip strength, practice with spring-loaded grip trainers. Friday also points out that working with free weights improves your grip while strengthening other muscles.

How to Be Uplifting

Of course, knowing *what* you need to do doesn't mean you know *how* to do it. You may know which muscles you need for lifting, but do you know how to pick things up in the most powerful way? There is a method—it's safe, effective and makes you look strong.

Face forward. The worst thing you can do is lift something, then turn around.

"You're almost certain to twist your body to change direction—and if you're carrying a heavy object, you could really hurt yourself," says Dr. Donkin. So before you lift, position your body so you're facing in the direction you want to go.

Lift with your legs. You've heard the admonition a thousand times, but good advice always bears repeating: If you're going to lift, lift with your legs. "So many guys just don't get it. They still bend down and yank an object up with their back muscles. Then they hurt," says Friday. Instead, think of your legs like the hydraulics on a forklift, lowering, stopping while you get your arms around the object, then raising up.

Get close. The closer your body is to the object you want to lift, says Dr. Donkin, the better your balance will be when you lift it—and the less likely you'll be to use those back muscles incorrectly.

Tighten your gut. "When patients have back problems, the problem often is that they don't have strong abdominals—and they're absolutely necessary when you're lifting or holding an item," Dr. Donkin says. So as you start to lift, tighten your stomach muscles—that will help support the lower back and ensure that it doesn't bear the brunt of the load.

Plant your feet. Keep your feet shoulder-width apart when you're lifting. If you put them close together, you're robbing yourself of a stable lifting base.

Go straight. When you bend to pick up an item, says Friday, bend at the knees, not the waist. As you stand, keep your back and neck straight.

Take your time. Despite what your in-grained competitive instincts tell you as you start to exert yourself, you're not in a race. So instead of acting like you're training for the Olympic Box-Lifting Team, take your sweet time. "The more you rush, the better the odds of hurting yourself," says Dr. Donkin.

Use your head. If something's too heavy—and you *know* when something's too heavy—get a pal to help you lift it. It doesn't mean you're not a man—it just means you're not a man who'll have to spend the next six weeks in traction.

Be a Stand-Up Guy

We spend years of our lives standing around. Waiting at the cash machine. Getting on line for the bus. Queuing for concert tickets. Sometimes being an upstanding guy is just plain frustrating.

It's also potentially damaging to your body. "Anytime you're standing upright, your body is carrying a constant load—your very own body weight. And if you stand in any one position for any length of time, eventually that's going to irritate your lower spine," says Dr. Scott Donkin, a chiropractor in Lincoln, Nebraska. But here are two quick ways to take a load off your back—even when you can't sit down.

Step up. If you're near an object that's six inches to a foot higher than where you're standing, put one foot up there. "It could be a book, a footstool, a ledge, a step—anything that's just a little bit higher than the floor," says Dr. Donkin. Not only will you strike a rakish pose, you'll also change your body position just enough so that the pressure's off your back.

Be shifty. When there's no handy step around, shift your body weight from foot to foot. Don't do it so often that you look like you have to go to the bathroom—once every five minutes ought to be enough.

Throwing a Harder Punch

You Could Be a Contender

Violence is the last resort, an admission of failure. You know this, you do: It's better to turn the other cheek, to talk your way out of a fight, to never raise your hand against your fellow man.

Problem is, the *other* guy may not know that, or worse, may not care. Remember one of the first lessons you learned in school: There's a bully on every playground, some moke who thinks with his fists, who enjoys picking a fight, and one of these days—nothing personal—he's going to pick it with you.

And it's against that day that we store in our heads a secret knowledge, a means of defending ourselves when all reason fails.

We know how to punch.

Think about it—even if you've never punched someone in your life, you know how to do it. And though you hope never to use it, a part of you wouldn't mind knowing how to make that punch even stronger.

Keys to Power

Even in a civilized world, punching is a handy thing to know. When the front door's jammed, the washing machine's on the blink or we want to vent some frustration on the heavy bag in the basement, we may feel it's time for a well-aimed blow. In those situations it's good to know how to punch with conviction—and how to do it without breaking a knuckle.

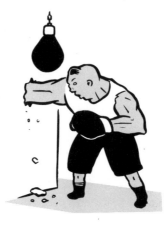

"The problem is most guys throw punches or push them at their opponent," says Joe Lewis, a former amateur world karate champ. As Lewis explains, when you throw a punch, you cock your hand back and hurl it forward like a baseball. "Not only are you telegraphing your move to an opponent, you're also bringing your shoulder too far over your hips—you lose balance and power," he says.

Pushing a punch isn't any better. "The problem there is you'll throw your shoulder forward first and lean forward at the waistline, basically pushing your fist into your opponent's face," Lewis says. "This leaves your legs out of the equation and that's bad—a good punch comes from your lower body."

The trick, world-class hitters agree, is to release the punch, to let it explode from your body. Here's how.

Make a commitment. Once you've decided to punch, says Lewis, don't have second thoughts. "There's an emotional component to punching that can be very powerful if you can control it," says the martial arts expert. "When you punch, you should have an emotional energy behind it, what we call conviction. The formula for punching is: Effort plus conviction equals substance. If you don't have substance, you don't have a punch."

Relax. The biggest problem with throwing an effective punch is channeling both the mental and emotional power of your entire body into a single fist. But if every muscle in your body is tense, your full punching power will never make it to your hand.

"Relaxing before a punch is the hardest thing to learn because there's so much emotion involved in punching," says David Lawrence, a former welterweight boxer and a trainer at Gleason's Boxing Gym in Brooklyn Heights, New York. "You have to detach the fear, the concern, or else refocus it into the punch. You can't worry about the damage you'll do or the retaliation or anything."

Shift your weight. Karate champ Lewis says punching power comes from your feet. "Basically, the secret is to shift your weight from your back foot to your front foot. The weight shift is controlled by your ankles—that's where the power's coming from." So practice shifting your weight from foot to foot. Have your weight resting on the heel of your back foot. Slowly transfer it from the heel to the ball of the rear foot, then to the heel of your front foot. "Feel the weight shifting, get comfortable with it. Then you'll be able to put your weight behind a punch," says Lewis.

Get your hips into the punch. From the weight shift, punching power transfers up the legs to your hips. "You have to keep your hips relaxed and learn to torque your hips, to swivel them as the weight is coming forward. Then you're going to bring your shoulder forward—the shoulder will follow the hip motion," Lewis says. Your arm should not be back behind you, but close at your side, elbow bent, fist ready. Because, at the end of that pivot, you'll release your punch.

Punch through the target. As your fist comes forward, pick a point about a foot behind your target and aim for it. "This technique is called punching through your opponent and it's very effective," says Lawrence. Otherwise, you lose power by trying to stop the punch right at the moment of contact. "You'll seize up without even thinking about it and lose a lot of speed and power," agrees Lewis. As you're punching through, extend your arm out, but don't lock it. "You lock your arm out and you can really hurt the elbow

joint—even if you miss," says Lawrence.

Recoil the spring. When you reach the end of your release, don't try to stop your arm. "Imagine your arm is like a rubber band. If you keep it loose and let momentum do the work, your arm will recoil back to the body. This is called snapping the punch and it can add power to the blow, too," Lawrence says.

A Knockout Workout

"When I'm training fighters, I have them focus more on technique than any kind of weight-lifting regimen," says former welterweight boxer and Gleason's Boxing Gym trainer David Lawrence. "In a fight, technique is always a better asset than strength."

Here are some exercises Lawrence recommends for his fighters. One note: When hitting the heavy bag and speed bag, be sure to wear bag gloves—which you can find in most sporting goods stores—for protection.

• *Shadowboxing:* A powerful aerobic exercise that gets your arms and legs moving, shadowboxing involves no tools other than your own body. "It's a mixture of moving around on your feet, shifting your weight back and forth and, literally, punching at the air," Lawrence says. Do five rounds—three minutes per round—of flat-out shadowboxing per day. "You'll work up a great sweat," says Lawrence.

• *Speed bag:* Punching a speed bag builds reaction time and eye-hand coordination. You can buy your own for less than $100, or call your local fitness club or YMCA and ask if they have one. "You want to try to get a good rhythm going. It takes time to learn," says Lawrence. Try to do three three-minute rounds with the speed bag per workout session.

• *Heavy bag:* Working out on the heavy bag strengthens wrists and upper arms and approximates the bulk of an opponent. You can hang a heavy bag in your basement and practice body strikes, as well as vent a little work-related frustration. Do five three-minute rounds.

Dancing the Night Away

Getting in the Groove

Fred Astaire, you're not—and John Travolta, you never want to be (at least not in his white-suited *Saturday Night Fever* incarnation). Yet between those two poles of the male dancing pantheon is an enviable position—that of the good dancer. And truth to tell, you wouldn't mind being there—a light-on-his-feet kind of guy, well-known for his ability to cut a rug.

Instead, it's more likely you'll cut out in the middle of an evening of dancing, suffering as much from exhaustion as from embarrassment. Meanwhile, your dance partner spins on like a whirling dervish, oblivious to your near cardiac arrest, your aching feet, your bruised ego.

Firing Up the Dance Machine

Dancing may not be viewed as the most masculine activity, but believe it or not, a little trip on the light fantastic can actually help your workout.

"There's a lot of movement. You're using muscles that are different from the ones you normally use," says Dan Downing, a power lifter—and an accomplished ballroom dancer—in Allentown, Pennsylvania. "I've been doing both for years and I love them. It's a strange combination, but they go well together." Lifting may tighten muscles, Downing says, but dancing helps keep those muscles supple and limber.

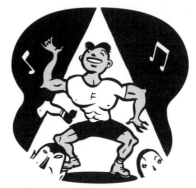

Well, that's one concern solved—you don't have to feel like a weenie when you hit the dance floor. But how to keep from *looking* like one?

"Dancing is very demanding—it can be as energetic an exercise as sprinting," says Dennis Rogers of Westfield, New Jersey, treasurer for the National Dance Council of America and a dance instructor for more than 40 years. And while dancing itself is a great cardiovascular exercise, Rogers says it doesn't hurt to be doing other cardiovascular and aerobic exercises. If anything, they'll make you a better dancer. "You see a lot of dancers at the competitive level who will do aerobics and other exercises. They're training for dancing," says Rogers.

We're not about to suggest you start sweatin' to the oldies every night so you can be a weekend dance machine, but you can improve your dancing—and your overall health—with just a few simple steps.

Teach yourself a lesson. Okay, as a man, you probably won't set foot in an aerobic dance class. But what about a ballroom dance class, like the muscular Mr. Downing, or a country line-dancing class? "Dance lessons are a great form of exercise—and it's something you can do with your partner, too," says Rogers.

Focus on your partner. One reason men are so tense on the dance floor is because they're self-conscious. On unfamiliar ground we're only too ready for people to start pointing and laughing. Worse yet, we're just waiting for some moussed-out lounge lizard to swagger onto the floor and begin spinning his partner—or maybe even yours—from one end of the room to the other, while we slouch off to the bar.

To solve this problem, repeat this simple phrase to yourself: To hell with everyone else.

"Don't worry about looking bad. Instead, pay attention to only one person—your partner," says Rogers. "I can tell you as a dance instructor that the more you focus on yourself and your partner, the better dancer you'll be. And the better you are, the less you'll care if other people are watching you."

Stay loose. Whatever the dancing venue, try to wear loose clothing. If you're country line-dancing, slap on a pair of relaxed-fit jeans. If you're at your brother's wedding, loosen your tie or make sure that cummerbund isn't too tight. "The more constricting the clothes, the less maneuverability you'll have. You'll get hot and wear out faster," says John Amberge of the Sports Training Institute.

Drink up. Whether you're under the blaring lights, caught in the press of gyrating bodies or gracefully gliding across the ballroom with your partner, it's only a matter of time before your body will start screaming for fluids. "If you don't drink water often, you'll eventually wear yourself out," says Rogers. "That's why at professional dance competitions, they have water stations set up all around the dance floor." So take a break every 10 or 15 minutes and slake that thirst with water. Try to keep alcoholic beverages to a minimum—alcohol will just make you even more dehydrated.

Take up aerobics. If you want to be a hot shot at the dance club, hit the health club first. Okay, so you're not the type to sign up for an aerobics class—include some other type of cardiovascular activity in your workout instead. "Stair-climbers, rowing machines, treadmills, stationary bicycles and cross-country skiers are all excellent aerobic tools that improve your cardiovascular health," Amberge says. Plus, they tone your legs and other crucial dancing muscles. Finally, you may be surprised to discover that the aerobic workout will do a lot more than help your dancing—it'll also improve your regular cardiovascular workout.

Put on Your Dancing Shoes

If you're not wearing the right shoes, dancing can be pretty bad for your feet, to say nothing of your dancing form. And you can't wear just any old thing when you dance. "Some shoes feel good until you try dancing in them," says dance instructor Dennis Rogers of Westfield, New Jersey. "People talk about wearing their dancing shoes—it's a good idea to have a pair."

Don't go out and ask your shoe salesman for a pair of dancing shoes, though—just pick a pair that has plenty of cushioning. "A hard-soled, stiff shoe is going to hurt, and it limits your agility," says Rogers. For casual dancing you'd be better off to go with a thick-soled walking shoe.

But what if it's a black-tie affair, and you have to wear the nicest-looking, least comfortable shoes you own? Or you're going out line-dancing and those cowboy boots are painful just to look at?

In that case, pad them yourself with insoles, which you can find in any drugstore and most supermarkets. "Just a little padding adds a lot of comfort, and it will show when you dance," says Rogers.

Stretch. Dance expert Rogers says professional dancers often stretch before competition. You probably should too—even if it's just a night of country swing dancing. If you haven't been dancing in a while and your legs and hips are feeling a little bit tight, spend about 15 minutes doing some basic total-body stretches, then concentrate on the lower body.

Not only will you dance better that night, you also won't feel so sore the next day. And when your partner suggests going out again the next night, you won't have to give her a song and dance about why you can't make it.

Holding a Baby

How to Raise Your Child Right

In the movie *When Harry Met Sally*, Meg Ryan and Billy Crystal's characters debate the trials and tribulations of child-rearing. Ryan's beef: that women only have a certain number of fertile years. "It's different for men," she says. "Charlie Chaplin had babies when he was 73."

"Yeah," Crystal shoots back, "but he was too old to pick 'em up."

That's the blessing and the curse of children: It's wonderful to pick them up and carry them around, but for a sedentary father it can be physical torture, too. If you don't have kids, you don't often realize the strength and stamina required by parenthood. As any self-respecting mom or dad can tell you, child-raising is a workout.

To give you non-dads an idea, cradle a bowling ball in one arm and carry it around the house for an hour. That's life with a few-month-old who will only go in the crib after being walked in circles by papa during an entire Beethoven symphony.

But the fun doesn't end there, because the little rug rat keeps getting bigger by the day. Now try spending an afternoon hauling the equivalent weight of a pre-walking toddler— say, a 20-pound sack of potatoes—and see how you feel. First, carry it in your arms. Then shift it from hip to hip. Put it on your shoulder, haul it on your back. Now try all of this while walking a mile or two. Starting to feel a little soreness in your wrists, your neck, your arms, your back? And you still have it easy—a bowling ball doesn't emit headache-inducing screams; a sack of potatoes is never going to throw up on you.

Child-rearing, on the other hand, is one great, big, messy, slapstick comedy. And if you don't want the joke to be on you, start spending some time building the strength and stamina you'll need to carry you through the trials of fatherhood.

Being a Firm Father

Raising a child is such a mental and emotional strain, it's easy to forget the wear and tear a tyrannical tyke can inflict on your poor old body. Kids want to be picked up. They want a piggyback ride. They want to be tossed in the air until they throw up. And your obligations are clear in this arena: Unless you want to abdicate your title as World's Greatest Dad, you're expected to perform these duties endlessly. You can spare yourself a lot of sprains and strains and evenings curled up with a heating pad if you just train your body to deal with the perils of parenting.

"As you get older and tend to be more sedentary, sudden bursts of physical activity"—such as being ambushed by a gang of five-year-old pirates—"can lead to muscle strains and injuries, especially in the back," says Roy Shephard, M.D., Ph.D., professor emeritus of applied physiology at the University of Toronto, Ontario. "That's why the older you get, the more important it is to incorporate as much vigorous activity as you can into your daily living."

Here are a few basic exercises to keep you going.

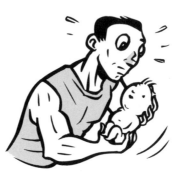

Flex before fun. As we get older, it gets harder to go from a seated position in the La-Z-Boy to all-out warfare with a junior G.I. Joe. So before you play, give your muscles a little play by stretching them, says Dr. Shephard. Just give yourself five minutes and focus on your lower back, shoulders and legs. The stretching will keep your muscles supple and prevent those nasty pulls and strains that come so easily while diving into an imaginary foxhole. If your kid is harping insistently at you, turn it into a game that he can play. Tell him to get down on the floor with you and play Simon Says.

Build a better back. As with any lifting and carrying—especially of wriggling, squirming objects like children—make sure your back is strong and limber enough to do the job, says Northwestern University strength and conditioning coach Jeff Friday. A good exercise for the back is the back extension. Weight-training exercises that help include the deadlift and the bent-over row. Be sure to do these slowly. "Take your time," admonishes Friday.

Work your abs. The abdominal muscles are an important foundation for all the carrying and roughhousing your other muscles do, and they do double-duty supporting the lower back, Friday says. So when you work out, be sure to do plenty of abdominal crunches.

Arm yourself. Whether you're wrestling in the rec room, tossing junior up in the air or warming up for the first of an infinite number of games of catch, you want your arms in good shape. Pennsylvania State University strength and conditioning coach Chip Harrison suggests biceps curls and tricep extensions.

Get a leg under you. Another trick to help you lift increasingly heavy objects—and support them for longer periods of time—is the leg crisscross, which strengthens the lower back. Sit on the floor with legs extended, slightly bent at the knees. Keeping your hands on the floor and knees bent, lift your feet a few inches off the floor. Now cross your left foot over your right foot, keeping a half-inch space between the two. Hold for a moment, then

---

Your Son, the Football

For fathers of newborns, few pastimes are as perversely enjoyable as the football hold, in which you handle your squealing infant like a pigskin—to the mutual enjoyment of both of you. Here's how you do it, advises University of Toronto Dr. Roy Shephard. Just make sure you don't fumble the ball.

Face up: Lie the infant on his back along the length of your arm. Cradle his head in your hand and tuck your elbow into your side, as though you were about to make a run for the goal line.

Face down: As the baby gets older, he will have enough strength to hold his head up while he lies on his tummy along your arm. Hold his shoulders and upper chest in your hand and let his legs straddle the crook of your elbow. Tuck your elbow into your side for extra support.

---

switch, crossing right over left. Do two sets of 12 to 15 reps.

Give your kids a leg up. Even with strong legs and a firm lower back, don't forget the basics of heavy lifting.

- Stand as close to the object, er, child as you can.
- Separate your feet to about shoulder-width apart.
- Bend at the knees—not the waist.
- Tighten your stomach muscles.
- Exhale as you lift.

Shoulder your responsibility. Finally, to prep for the inevitable piggyback rides, and also to support your throwing arm, work the shoulders. Harrison suggests lateral raises and military presses. If you can work these lifts into your weekly regimen, all the hours you'll spend fooling around with your kids will seem like child's play.

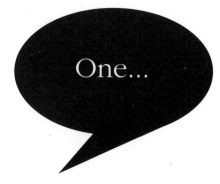

Part Five

The Perfect Exercise

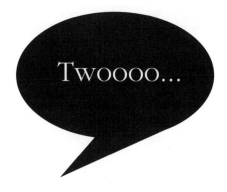

The Perfect Exercise

Push-Ups

The push-up is the elder statesman of exercises, a classic that never goes out of style. Push-ups hearken back to a time before circuit training, before weights. Back then, when a man wanted to strengthen his arms, shoulders and chest, he did it using only his body against the force of gravity—it was literally him against the world.

No wonder, then, that in an age of perfectly balanced fitness routines and gyms filled with ergonomically calibrated weight-training devices, we still include the push-up in our workouts. "There are certainly plenty of weighted exercises that work the chest and arm muscles equally well, but you can do a push-up anywhere, any time," says Steven McCaw, Ph.D., associate professor of biomechanics at Illinois State University in Normal.

Now drop and give me 20.

Get down. Position your body at about a 45-degree angle to the floor, with your weight supported only by your palms and your toes. Your palms should be flat on the floor, shoulder-length apart. Keep your elbows slightly bent, not locked. Your fingers should be pointing forward, your feet together. Your legs, back and neck should be in a straight line, with your face down. Looking up places strain on your neck.

Push yourself. Slowly lower yourself until your chest is nearly touching the floor. Elbows are completely bent. Your back and legs should still be straight. Now slowly push yourself back to the starting position—that's one.

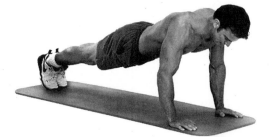

The ⬆ next level

One-handed push-ups aren't for beginners, says Illinois State University's Dr. Steven McCaw. "You have to have very strong arms and shoulders—to say nothing of good balance—otherwise you could seriously injure yourself."

Here's how you do a one-handed push-up.

Place your right hand on the floor and twist your body sideways. Place your left hand behind your back. If you need to, put your left foot sideways on the floor for balance. Only the toes and ball of your right foot should be touching the floor. Now push off with your arm—when it's straight and supporting your body weight, you're ready to begin.

Slowly lower yourself down until you're about four to five inches from the floor. As you go down, you may place your free hand on your hip for more balance. Now push back up to the starting position. Do three to five reps, then switch arms. Slowly work your way up to more reps.

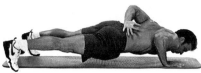

The Perfect Exercise

Crunches

If your abdominal muscles have become flab-dominals, you need to sit up and do something about it—with the exercise known as a crunch.

Forget the traditional, and woefully inefficient, sit-ups of junior-high gym classes. They can injure your neck and lower back and put too much stress on your hip-flexor muscles. Worst of all, they barely work the abdominals. Crunches, meanwhile, target those gut muscles exclusively and can get your abs in fab shape.

"To make a crunch effective, you really have to think about the muscles you want to work," says Ellington Darden, Ph.D., a fitness expert and strength-training researcher in Gainesville, Florida, and author of *Living Longer Stronger*. To find your abdominal muscles, try this: Sit down, lean forward and push your rib cage down toward your navel. Feel those muscles? They're your target.

Assume the position. Grab a handy exercise mat and lie down, keeping your back as flat as possible—arching strains the back and takes the load off the abs. Fold your arms across your chest and keep them there. If you lift your arms during a crunch, momentum—not your abs—does all the work. Keep your knees bent at a 45-degree angle, about three to four inches apart. Feet should be flat on the floor and no more than six or so inches from your butt—any farther and you'll start arching your back.

Variation: For additional resistance, cup your hands behind your ears when doing the crunch. Just don't lock your hands behind your neck or use them to pull up your head.

Sit up. Now it's time to crunch, so keep your neck relaxed and tuck your chin toward your chest—this minimizes strain. Slowly curl your torso upward. Your shoulder blades should be curled slightly up off the mat, no more than six inches off the floor. Your lower back should never leave the mat. Don't let your knees touch as you go through the crunch—that's cheating. And watch your heels—pushing down on them causes calves and hip-flexors to do all the work. Keep your movements smooth and controlled. After just a few crunches you should start to feel a burning sensation as though you'd done a dozen old-fashioned sit-ups.

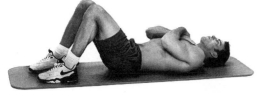

The ⬆ next level

You say your abs are fabulous, not flab-ulous, Captain Crunch? Then it's time to take your medicine—as in medicine ball. To do a power crunch, fitness expert Dr. Ellington Darden says to clutch a weight to your chest—a medicine ball or five- or ten-pound weight plate will do fine—and *then* see how many reps you can do.

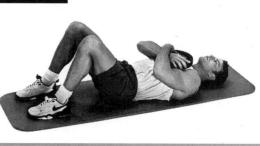

The Perfect Exercise

Jumping Jacks

Before the stair-climbing machine, before the NordicTrack, before the full-body aerobics workout, there was that cornerstone of calisthenics: the jumping jack. From gym class to football practice to boot camp, it has been a part of most guys' lives. But the exercise does more than make you feel like one of the Village People as you bob up and down. It's an activity that gets your pulse racing and, more important, gets you warmed up for those weights you're about to lift.

Unlike the push-up or the sit-up, jumping jacks are primarily a cardiovascular calisthenic—they benefit the heart and lungs far more than specific muscle groups like the pecs or the abs.

"The idea behind jumping jacks is to get the system up and running, to be a warm-up before a more strenuous workout," says Illinois State University's Dr. Steven McCaw. "But you need to be a little careful—it's an exercise that's deceptively hard on the body." According to the experts, swinging your arms and legs through a quick range of leaping motions can cause a lot of stress to joints, especially shoulders and hips.

"That's why you don't want to do jumping jacks with, say, wrist and ankle weights strapped on. When you swing your arms or legs, the weights at the end of your limbs generate a great deal of momentum and will become really heavy, which could cause an injury," warns Chip Harrison, strength and conditioning coach at Pennsylvania State University in State College. "Instead, you should just rely on your own weight and the vigor

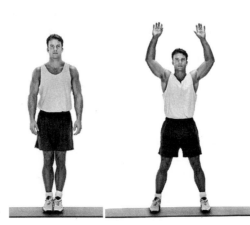

of the exercise to warm you up. When they're done correctly, jumping jacks are good warm-up exercises," Harrison adds. "They're the kind of activity you want to do before you launch into heavy flexibility work or before you go out running."

A few sets of jumping jacks can be as pulse-raising as a quick stint in an aerobics class—only you don't need to have a sense of rhythm. Or wear spandex. Here's how to get jumping, Jack.

Make your stand. Start with your arms at your sides, feet together, back straight. To work your calves out a little more, stand up on your toes. Inhale before you jump.

Jump-start your workout. Jump a few inches off the floor, bringing your arms in a wide circular path over your head. Exhale when your hands are up. If you want to clap your hands at the top of the motion—like your gym teacher probably taught you—go right ahead. One word of caution: Clap lightly. Smacking your hands together hard could damage your shoulders over an extended period of time. As you raise your arms, spread your legs until your feet are a little wider than shoulder-width apart—that's the position you want to land in. To make it easier on your hip joints, try splitting your legs forward and backward, instead of side to side. For a mild warm-up, do 20 at a moderate speed.

Variation: To keep things interesting, try varying the move by raising your arms forward and backward, skipping with your feet like you're jumping rope, or crossing your feet as you bring them together to improve agility and balance.

"No matter what variation you do, remember to maintain safe technique," Harrison says. "You don't want to explain to your buddies that you hurt yourself in the gym—doing jumping jacks."

The Perfect Exercise

Pull-Ups

Just this once, think of yourself as one big dumbbell. Pull-ups are a simple exercise that will power up the shoulders with minimal equipment. All you need is a sturdy chinning bar that lets you hang about six inches off the ground and your body to supply the weight. Chinning bars are standard equipment at gyms and playgrounds, or you can pick one up at a sporting goods store and mount it at home in a door frame or in the basement.

"Basically, a pull-up will increase the strength in the shoulder muscles, the upper arms and the upper-back muscles," says Bob Viau, a Baltimore phys- ical therapist and trainer. "Your body weight determines how much you will progress." If you want more of a workout from your pull-ups, you can always add weight to your body, Viau notes. Wrap a chain around your waist and hang a weight from it. Or try ankle weights.

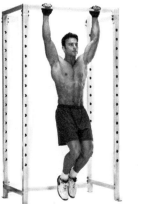

If you're new to pull-ups, try doing just two or three at first and see how you feel the next day. If your muscles are sore, take an extra day's rest before resuming. If you're having trouble completing a pull-up, keep trying until you go all the way up and down. That full range of motion makes the exercise more effective, Viau says.

As with any weight lifting, pull-ups should be done with a steady motion. "A lot of people feel that getting that last rep in and jerking themselves up is a benefit," Viau says. "It's not: You could sustain an injury."

Get a grip. Grasp the chinning bar, placing your hands 18 to 20 inches apart, palms facing away. When you're hanging, your feet should be about 6 inches off the ground.

Pull up. With a slow, steady motion, pull yourself up until your chin is higher than the bar. Then lower yourself to the starting position. Exhale on your way up, and inhale on your way down. Don't let your body swing. Try to keep your back slightly arched backward.

The ⬆ next level

If standard pull-ups aren't enough of a challenge, try this.

With your hands still facing palms out, widen your grip on the chinning bar to 32 to 34 inches apart. This increases the degree of difficulty and works the upper lats. Using a slow and steady motion, pull yourself up and try to touch the back of your neck to the bar. Then lower yourself to the starting position. Breathe out on the way up, and breathe in on the way down.

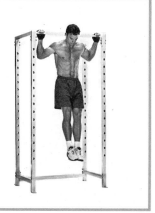

The Perfect Exercise

Jumping Rope

If you want to burn fat, boost your cardiovascular capacity, tone muscle and improve agility and rhythm, you could sink a thousand bucks into a fancy home gym. Or you could buy a jump rope.

A 165-pound man jumping rope can burn 14.2 calories in a minute, or 852 calories an hour. That's more than jogging or cycling.

Ken M. Solis, M.D., author of the book *Ropics: The Next Jump Forward in Fitness*, offers these pointers.

- Give yourself enough rope. When you stand in the middle, the ends of the handles should just reach your armpits.
- Land on the balls of your feet, not your

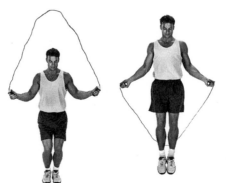

toes or heels. Then roll back toward your heels and push off again. Jump only an inch or less off the ground. Wood, vinyl tile or low carpeting makes the best jumping surfaces.

- Your wrists and forearms should do the turning, not your shoulders. Arms stay at your sides, with elbows tucked in.
- Wear well-padded cross-trainers or aerobics shoes. Running shoes generally won't do.

Here's how to do basic rope-jumping.

Get in the swing. Start with a handle in each hand and the rope behind you, feet together. Use your wrists to swing the rope up and over your head. Keep your hands at waist-level and your elbows tucked in.

Jump. As the rope nears your feet, jump up an inch to let the rope pass underneath. Land on the balls of your feet. Aim for about 130 skips per minute—or just over two skips a second.

The ⌂ next level

When you're ready for a little variation in your rope-jumping, try the jog step. As with the basic jump, begin with the rope behind you. Bend your knee to raise your right foot behind you about six inches. Start turning, and as the rope approaches, hop on your left foot to let the rope pass under while the right foot remains raised. Hop on the left foot for several jumps, then switch sides by jumping up with your left foot and landing on your right, this time raising the left foot. When you're comfortable with the one-foot hop on each side, lower the number of hops on each foot until you're switching back and forth with each jump.

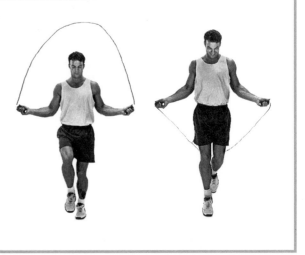

The Perfect Exercise

Bicycling

Going for a long, weekend bike ride is a great way to relax and get away from the pressures of the office and home. But if you don't learn to relax on the bike, you're not going to get very far, says training expert Fred Matheny.

"So many people ride with a really tense upper body and a death grip on the bars," says Matheny, fitness and training editor of *Bicycling* magazine and author of *Weight Training for Cyclists*. "And they use up a lot of energy that way."

If you want to use your bike to get fit, first you have to make sure you fit your bike. A visit to your local bicycle shop, particularly one that features the Fit Kit or the Serotta Sizecycle, is a good place to start. Once the proper adjustments are made to your bike, it's not just a matter of climbing on and happily pedaling off. From head to toe, your position on the bike largely determines how quickly you fatigue. Here are the basics, according to Matheny.

Look up. Because of fatigue, many bikers ride with their heads down. While that gives you a splendid view of your front hub, it does create one minor problem: You're liable to run into a parked car or a wall because you can't see where you're going. So remember to always keep your head up.

Back down. Your shoulders should be relaxed, and your back should be flat—or as close to it as your body's natural shape allows. This actually helps you breathe more efficiently by

opening up your chest cavity. If your back on the bike resembles Marty Feldman's Igor in *Young Frankenstein*, it could be a sign that your bicycle's top tube-stem combination is too short.

Bend your elbows. The old stiff-arm may come in handy for football running backs trying to break a tackle, but it can cause fatigue and increase your chances of crashing on a bike. If your arms are stiff, any bumps in the road will send shock waves straight through your body. It also severely limits your ability to steer. Concentrate on keeping your elbows slightly bent. This will allow your arms to absorb road shocks and put you in position to maneuver quickly when needed.

Flutter your fingers. For cruising speed, your hands should be on top of the levers. This position offers the best of all worlds: It's reasonably aerodynamic, provides stability and allows easy access to the brake levers. To accelerate, move your hands forward on the drops—the lower arms of the handlebars. For moderate uphill climbs, try moving your hands to the upper bends. And remember to ease up on the death grip. With your palms on the handlebar, occasionally flutter your fingers to stay relaxed.

Sit and slide. Once the saddle is positioned correctly, you should primarily be seated in the center for long rides. If you need a sudden burst of speed, you'll slide forward onto the tip of the saddle. If you're climbing a long, steady hill, you'll slide to the back, which cuts down on pedaling cadence but generates more power, Matheny says.

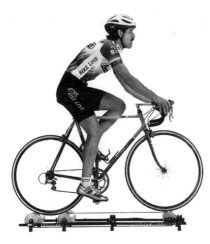

Have a ball. The ball of your foot should be directly over the pedal axle. If it's too far behind the axle, you can wind up with an Achilles tendon strain.

The Perfect Exercise

Running

It doesn't get much simpler than running. As the old saying goes, you just put one foot in front of the other. But precisely *where* you put that front foot can make all the difference between running injury-free and being hobbled by leg pain.

"I hate to be negative, but when people err, they tend to bounce off the ground too high and they tend to overstride," says former U.S. Olympic marathoner Jeff Galloway, who has worked with thousands of runners and is author of the best-selling *Galloway's Book on Running.*

When your lead foot strikes the road, it should be directly under your knee. If your foot is hitting the ground in front of your knee, it's as if you're hitting the brakes with each stride. If you want to know if you're overstriding, take the sock test, devised by Budd Coates, a national-class distance runner and *Men's Health* magazine fitness consultant. While running, simply look down as your lead foot hits the ground. If you can see your sock, you're overstriding. If you're running with the proper form—so that your leg is at a 90-degree angle when your heel meets the road—you won't be able to see your sock.

Our running experts offer these other basic tips that will help you run longer and stronger.

Warm up, stretch out. Increase your flexibility and efficiency, as well as avoid injury, by first warming up before your run with a few minutes riding on a stationary bike, jumping rope or simply walking briskly. Then end your run with a cooldown period of slower movement, and follow up with a few minutes of gentle stretching.

Stay fluid. During your running motion, concentrate on lifting your knee just enough to let your leg swing forward naturally. Again, the idea is to direct your energy into moving forward—not bouncing up-and-down.

Be hip. Keep your hips relaxed, your butt tucked in and your pelvis slightly forward. This will keep your center of gravity slightly in front of you, making it easier for your legs to propel your body forward.

Go straight. Don't let your upper body twist from side to side while you're running. Remember, the idea is to move forward. Keep your feet pointed basically straight ahead—not twisted to either side.

Relax. Keep your shoulders and upper arms relaxed, with your shoulders directly above your hips. Your elbows should be close to the body, flexed at about 90 degrees through the full range of the armswing. Your hands should be loose, but not limp.

Heads up! Make a conscious effort to fix your eyes on the horizon. Keeping your head up and your eyes forward will help increase your stride length and also help you run more efficiently.

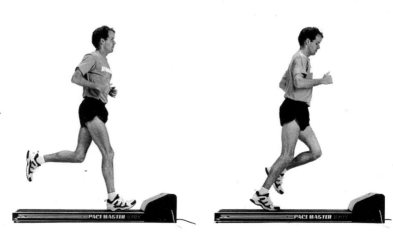

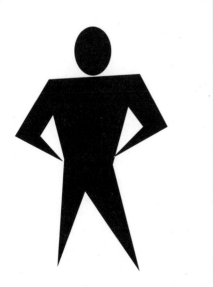

Part Six

Real-Life Scenarios

Power Routines
It's time to put it all together. A blueprint to help you achieve your personal goals.

Quest for the Best
They've been willing to pay the price to be powerfully fit. How do they stay in such great shape?

You Can Do It!
Different lives, different careers—but one thing in common: These typical men have made themselves powerfully fit. You can, too.

Power Routines

It's time to get with the program. Whether you want bulging biceps or limber legs, here's the blueprint for a better body. Choose the plan that best achieves your individual goals.

Health and Fitness Programs

Grow Stronger, Live Longer

So you're sitting there thinking to yourself, "I can get fit anytime I want ... I'm just not quite sure where to start."

Smart lad.

No, seriously. You can't just walk into a weight room, start lifting and expect that you're going to get a healthy, well-muscled physique. That's insane—you'll end up with a pulled muscle first, or worse, a heart attack. No, every coach needs a game plan, every general needs a strategy and every body—yours, too—needs a basic fitness scheme, a simple formula that will slowly start you on the path to the level of fitness you've always felt you deserved (if only you knew where to start). It involves nutrition, cardiovascular power, flexibility and, of course, a weight-training routine that you can grow with. Now you're thinking, if you had a program that covered all that, you would be able to get fit anytime you wanted.

Well, here it is.

Fueling for Fitness

Before you even lift your first weight, you need to take stock of what you've been lifting to your lips.

"Nutrition is sometimes

the forgotten link in the exercise equation. A lot of men don't pay much attention to what they eat," says Bob Arnot, M.D., medical correspondent for CBS News and author of *Dr. Bob Arnot's Guide to Turning Back the Clock.* And that's too bad, says Dr. Arnot, because the first step to fitness is figuring out what fuel is going to keep your body revving like a super-charged muscle car, and avoiding the stuff that could gum up your engine. Here's a quick primer.

Fend off fat. Nothing keeps you out of the gym like fat. Eat too much of it, and you won't feel like getting off the couch, much less displaying your larded self in a gym full of people in various stages of physical betterment. But besides being an impediment to sculpting the ideal body, fat's also a furtive killer. Saturated fats—the kind you'll find in steaks and cheeses and other foods you love—clog arteries and cause heart disease, the biggest killer of men. But you can increase your odds of avoiding heart disease with just a few modifications to your eating style. Start by reading labels and watching your intake of red meat and dairy products.

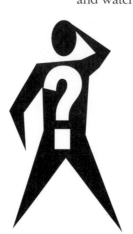

Prep with protein. Although you should go easy on meat and dairy products, it's okay to have a cut of lean meat, a glass of milk or a cup of yogurt once in a while. Reason is, to build new muscle, your body needs protein. Favorite lower-fat protein sources include fish, poultry, beans, low-fat yogurt and skim milk.

Become a carbo hold.

When you're on a regular fitness regimen, your body needs efficient fuel to help power you through your workout. No food is more efficient to the human body than carbohydrates. Eat them, especially after a workout. You'll find carbs in most grain foods, pastas and legumes.

Tap water's power. Experts say most of us don't drink enough water—a fact that can prove dangerous during a workout. "If you don't stay hydrated during a workout, you'll start losing power fast, then you won't be exercising effectively," says Budd Coates, *Men's Health* magazine fitness consultant. So try to drink about eight to ten glasses of water during the day, and keep a water bottle with you when you work out. Take a drink between sets, even if you don't feel thirsty. "If you wait until you're thirsty, it's too late—you're already losing power," says Coates.

Warming Up

Going straight from the couch to the weight bench is too big a jump for any man, no matter how physically fit he is. As a proper prep for working out, you need some light physical activity to prime your heart and other muscles. In other words, you need to warm up.

"You don't want to work a cold muscle," says Chip Harrison, strength and conditioning coach at Pennsylvania State University in State College. "That's why a five- to ten-minute warm-up is so important—it gets blood flowing to the muscles, increases their core temperature and makes them easier to work. If you try to lift weights without warming up, you could injure yourself."

A warm-up also can serve another

Are You Nimble, Jack?

Okay, these factors are not exactly indicators of brute strength, but can you imagine a tennis pro with lousy reflexes or a basketball star with little hand-eye co-ordination? Let's see how nimble—and quick—you really are. Charles Kuntzleman, Ed.D., associate professor in the Division of Kinesiology at the University of Michigan in Ann Arbor, suggests the following:

Ruler catch: To see how your reaction time measures up, ask a friend to dangle a ruler between your thumb and index finger and drop it without warning. In the ready position the zero end of the ruler should be just between your fingers. Hold your fingertips close, but not touching. When the ruler drops, catch it and check the inch-mark where your fingers land. You get to try three times and use your best score. Zero to six inches is good. More than six inches means your reaction time needs work.

Shooting baskets: Anybody can talk trash on the basketball court. The real question is: Can you shoot it? First, warn your boss that you're actually doing something extremely important—checking your hand-eye coordination. Then position your office chair ten feet from a standard trash can. Crumple a sheet of paper into a ball and take ten shots. Six or more baskets, good. Five or less, needs work.

---

important function by exercising the heart and lungs and improving your cardiovascular fitness, which will give you the heart and lung power to stay in the game.

If you're short on time, a 5- or 10-minute warm-up will get your body ready to lift weights. But if you do have the time, take about 15 or 20 minutes and turn your warm-up into a cardiovascular workout. Here's how.

Take the "A" train. When most guys hear the word "aerobics," they immediately think of fat women sweating to the oldies with Richard Simmons. But aerobics is far more than bad dancing to worse music. It's a classification of physical activity that includes many of your favorite sports.

"Aerobic activity is basically anything that gets your arms and legs pumping, gets your heart beating faster and gets you moving and breathing in a continuous, rhythmic way," Coates says. The most common aerobic warm-ups include stair-climbing, running, cycling, even swimming. Choose the one *you* like best.

Take it easy. When you warm up, be careful not to overheat.

"The point is to prepare your body to do a heavier exercise, not to wear it out," Harrison says. Make sure your warm-up exercise isn't so strenuous that you can't breathe normally.

Train your heart. With any warm-up it's a good idea to find the ideal training zone for your heart. "Generally, the training zone is 60 to 75 percent of the maximum heart rate for your age," says Coates. Most gyms have a handy chart you can use to find your training rate, but you can figure it out on your own. Just subtract your age from 220 and multiply that number by 0.6. That gives you the low end of your training zone. You can figure the high end by subtracting your age from 220 and multiplying that number by 0.75. If you don't want to do the math, just check the chart on page 5. Twenty minutes is the minimum time experts say you should work out in that zone. "But anything is better than nothing," says Coates. The longer you can keep yourself in the zone, the better your cardiovascular health will be.

Get Fit Now

Do three sets of these exercises. The first set should be about 12 reps of a moderate weight; the second set should be 8 reps of a heavier weight. Your last set should be 4 reps of the heaviest weight you can lift. Be sure to rest about two minutes between each set. Now start pumping!

Muscle Group	Compound Exercise	Specific Exercise
Legs	Squats or Leg Presses	Leg Extensions, Leg Curls
	Seated or Standing Calf Presses	
Chest and Arms	Bench Presses	Fly Presses, Triceps Presses
Shoulders and Upper Body	Overhead or Military Presses	Lateral Raises, Shoulder Shrugs, Standing Rows

Making Muscle

Now that you're fine-tuning your body with a proper diet and a good warm-up, it's time for the real work—the weight training. You don't have to try power lifting right off the bat—you have plenty of time to work your way up to Mr. Universe level. If you're just starting out, you want to have a basic lifting routine that's going to tone you and build muscle. The chart above lists 11 exercises that, when done correctly, will make you powerfully fit. Make sure you have at least 48 hours rest between weight-lifting sessions. A quick note before you hit the bench: If you do all the exercises listed, you're looking at roughly an 80-minute workout. It's time well-spent, but we know that you won't always have it. When you're pressed, stick with the compound (those that involve two or more joints) exercise for each muscle group—that will only take you about 20 minutes.

Start light. Don't try to show off your first day in the gym. Begin with light weights, ones you can handle comfortably. "Recommendations for beginning weight-lifting levels are dependent upon the size and fitness level of the individual," Coates says. Use the lighter weights for your initial two or three progressive workouts.

Build a pyramid. You can gradually increase the amount of weight you use with a training system known as pyramid lifting.

"Basically, all that means is you exercise each major muscle group of your body, with three sets. The first set is about 12 reps of the most weight you can lift for that number of reps. Then you rest for two to three minutes. Each set after that, you want to do one-third fewer reps of more weights," Coates says. So for your second set, do 8 reps of the heaviest weight you can manage. On your last set you'll do just 4 reps of the most you can lift. "And I mean the most. After 4 reps you shouldn't be able to do 5 or 6. Overloading the muscles that way is what will really build stronger muscle," says Coates.

Increase your compound interest. For each muscle group do one compound exercise—something that works the group as a whole—and two specific lifts that target components of the muscle group. In the case of your legs, Coates suggests squats or leg presses as your compound exercise. To work specific leg muscles, do leg extensions and leg curls or either a standing or seated calf press.

Peg your legs first. When you work the muscle groups, some experts suggest starting with the legs.

"People generally dislike legwork. They always want to jump right in and do bench presses. I say do the legs first. That way you're working your largest muscle groups while you're fresh. If you don't like working the legs, it's over with. In fact, I like to move the chest exercises to the back of the workout. That way you're working toward the exercises that many people think are the most fun," Harrison says.

Ride the bench. Now, for your chest and arms. "The bench press is the obvious compound exercise," says Coates. "Then, to work specific muscles, you'll probably want to do a fly press and a tricep press."

Shoulder the burden. Finally, spend some time working your upper back and shoulders. Do an overhead or military press for your compound exercise. And if you own a weight belt, this is the time to wear it. Overhead exercises can hyperextend the back, and a weight belt can help prevent that. Don't wear it for the rest of your workout, otherwise you'll come to rely on it—and not your own muscles—too much. For your specific exercises try lateral raises, shoulder shrugs and standing rows.

Playing It Cool

Seems like a man's workout is never done. Even after all that hard lifting, it's not time to hit the showers yet.

"After a workout most guys just want to get out of there. But if you leave without stretching or cooling down, your muscles are going to contract too much. Not only will you be incredibly sore the next day, you'll start losing range of motion in the joints and muscles," Coates warns.

So take ten minutes to cool off, stretch out and prep your body for the next workout. Follow these guidelines.

Tread lightly. Make sure the cooldown is low-key. "If you're on a treadmill for your cooldown, you don't want to be running. Set it at a brisk walking level for a few minutes. The idea is to be slowing down the amount of physical activity, not starting up another exercise," says Coates.

Stretch out. To avoid lurching through the office looking like Quasimodo the next day because of tight muscles, do some simple stretches for your arms, back and legs. Focus also on your shoulders and triceps, as well as your lower back, hips, groin and hamstrings.

Power Programs

Paying Bulk Rate for Muscles

Go to any gym, and odds are you'll find full-length mirrors in the weight room. Granted, it's important for weight lifters to check their form while they pump. But let's be honest: Guys are essentially vain, and so what they're really looking at are the fruits of their hard labor. They want to see how good they look.

And there's absolutely nothing wrong with that. In fact, looking better is a prime motivator for many men who lift weights.

So in this chapter we're going to tell you how to build massive muscles. We're also going to teach you how to develop explosive power and strength. In fact, both goals are achieved through the same basic weight-lifting approach, says Wayne W. Campbell, Ph.D., an applied physiologist at Noll Physiological Research Center at Pennsylvania State University in University Park.

But first, a few warnings for those who want to bodybuild for the looks. It should be stated up front that not everyone can look like Mr. Universe. Nor is that necessarily a healthy goal.

"Society is so pegged with how you look. That could be your motivation, but it could be your downfall, too," warns Laura A. Gladwin, a fitness consultant, lecturer and owner of L.G.A. Fitness Consulting and Training in Brea, California. "Only 5 percent of men genetically have the ability to become an Arnold Schwarzenegger, and many stars are put together surgically or chemically."

Plus, if you think you'll be scoring babes with your inflated muscles, get a reality check. Surveys show that women in general are not into big, bulky guys. Yes, they want you trim and strong. But

rippling and bulging? Uh-uh.

Also, understand that bodybuilding takes a lot of time. It entails short spurts of brutal lifting intertwined with long periods of standing around while muscles recover. If you are to do bodybuilding right, plan on spending many hours a week in the gym. Is this a sacrifice you want to make?

All that said, there's plenty of good in bodybuilding. If done right, it can be completely healthy and immensely satisfying. That's why so many men are doing it. "Weight lifting now is universal. Within the last 30 years it's gone from being a subculture to mainstream," says Peter Lemon, Ph.D., professor of applied physiology at Kent State University in Kent, Ohio, and an avid lifter and expert in hypertrophy (muscle growth).

And no matter how resistant your body is to bulking up with muscle, you are guaranteed to benefit at least some by power training. Since the average guy's muscle fibers can balloon up to 40 percent in size, there's plenty of opportunity for everyone to improve.

"Even if you never look like Arnold, you'll be gaining mass and looking better," Gladwin says. "The most important thing is that you're exercising and feeling better about yourself."

Going to Mass

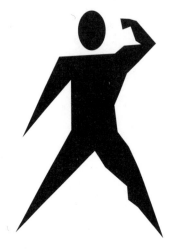

The right training for gaining strength and size boils down to two simple concepts: lifting the heaviest loads you can and eating an intensely focused, higher-calorie diet, Dr. Lemon says.

Even small fry can become big guys. A study in the Netherlands showed that small-framed men gained 14 percent more strength after a 12-week, twice-a-week weight-lifting program—the same gain as their beefier counterparts in the study.

The difference between weight lifting for general health and weight lifting for mass and power is like the difference between jogging for fun and running competitively: The basic movements are the same, but the intensity is drastically different. In normal workouts you tear down muscle fiber by lifting light to moderate weights. The muscle then grows stronger and slightly larger as it repairs itself. When you're lifting for mass, you shred muscle fiber more thoroughly because you're lifting heavier weights. Since you're adjusting your diet at the same time, you're feeding the muscle, thus firing up its growth and strength gains.

"Because you're breaking down your muscles so much when you lift for mass, you'll be very sore at first," says Steve Willard, head athletic trainer at Northwestern University in Evanston, Illinois. "But as your body accommodates, you'll get less and less sore, and you'll see the gains you want."

Power Foods

If your goal is to bulk up, training with heavy weights alone won't do the trick. Your muscles develop a voracious appetite, and they won't grow the way you want unless they're fed properly.

That means carbohydrates and proteins. Carbs offer energy for training, while proteins give you the raw materials for muscle growth. "Nutrition is critical. If you're trying to build mass, you'll need extra energy," Dr. Lemon says. "And without the right diet, you won't be seeing the results you want." As for protein, you'll need

Raging against Steroids

Anabolic steroids are a synthetic version of the male sex hormone, testosterone. They build muscle tissue and are prescribed by doctors to people whose bodies have atrophied because of illness or injury. Unfortunately, thanks to a black market and blind ambition, steroids are abused by some bodybuilders and other athletes wanting to build muscle fast.

Steroids are safe and have limited side effects when prescribed by a physician. Abusing steroids, however, can put your physical and mental health at risk. Abusers can experience drastic mood swings, including depression or uncontrolled aggression, called 'roid rage. They may also develop extreme acne, impotence, rashes and, in the long term, heart disease, liver tumors and testicle shrinkage. Sometimes, they die.

"If you're using steroids, your muscle is fake. It's phony. It's a shortcut," says Isaac Nesser of Scottdale, Pennsylvania, the Guinness world-record-holder for the largest chest and biceps. "Steroid users want something overnight. It's like our society—we're a now-or-never society. No one wants to work hard at their goals."

Nesser knows hard work. He's pumped his chest to an amazing 74$\frac{1}{16}$ inches and his biceps to a staggering 29 inches by spending upwards of six hours a day in the gym, seven days a week.

"And I'm completely drug-free and proud of it. I worked my butt off to have the biggest chest and arms in the world," Nesser says.

about four grams per every five pounds of body weight, daily, for best results, Dr. Lemon says. So if you weigh 150 pounds, you'll need about 120 grams of protein a day to maximize your muscle-building. That's as much as you'd get by having two large hard-boiled eggs and an eight-ounce glass of skim milk for breakfast, a six-ounce can of tuna and a glass of milk for lunch and a dinner consisting of a three-ounce serving of white turkey meat with a hearty cup of canned bean chili that's been fortified with one-half cup of boiled soybeans.

"Bear in mind that we've surveyed people and found it's common for them to eat more protein than they need," Dr. Lemon says. "So most guys won't need to increase protein. If you do, watch your water intake, because increasing protein too much can dehydrate you."

As for carbs, aim for 11 to 13 grams per 5 pounds of body weight, says Dr. Lemon. That means a 150-pound man should consume 330 to 390 grams of carbs a day, or about as much as you'd get in 2¾ cups of Wheatena and two bananas for breakfast, a baked potato and a six-ounce serving of dried pears for lunch and two cups of enriched spaghetti and one cup of lima beans for dinner.

"Many people who start a weight-lifting program are not consuming enough carbohydrates. Carbohydrates are the major fuel for training," Dr. Lemon says. Here are other tips from the experts on watching your diet for muscle gain.

Pump up the calories. As you gain muscle mass, you'll need to increase your total calorie consumption as well. It takes about 2,500 extra calories to build a pound of muscle. As for exactly how many extra calories you'll need, that'll take some experimenting because there's no secret formula. "If your goal is to gain more muscle, monitor your body weight and eat enough calories to keep it stable," says Dr. Campbell, "that way you'll be losing fat mass as you add muscle." Also, if you've been gaining weight slowly for months, weight training can help slow the rate of weight gain by building calorie-hungry muscle without depositing more fat, he adds.

Enjoy the snack attack. Eat healthy snacks whenever you're hungry. Your body knows best, and it'll tell your stomach to tell you that your muscles need nourishment. Healthy snacks include fruit, vegetables and grains, like breads. A couple of bananas and a hunk of pumpernickel might provide the energy and nutrients needed to build the muscle you want, says Dr. Campbell.

The Warm-Up

If you've ever been to a symphony, you've heard that awful cacophony the musicians make warming up. But without the warm-up, they wouldn't sound nearly as good for the real show. It's like that with weight lifting.

"Warming up increases the core temperature of your muscles and gets your cardiorespiratory system ready to respond to the exercises to follow," says John Graham, director of the Human Performance Center at the Allentown Sports Medicine and Human Performance Center in Allentown, Pennsylvania, whose clientele includes international champion athletes.

Graham, who is also a certified strength and conditioning specialist and certified United States Weight Lifting Federation Club Coach, suggests warming up with five or ten minutes of aerobic exercise, like jogging or cycling on a stationary bike, followed by ten minutes of total stretching, including your upper body. Then, he says, do one or two warm-up sets before you lift, using 60 percent of the weight you'll be working out with. For example, if you're bench-pressing 200 pounds, your warm-up set will be 10 to 12 reps at 120 pounds. This gives you time to mentally prepare for the heavier weight, while prepping your muscles for the upcoming load.

Sculpting a New You

We said before that power programs work much like other weight-lifting programs, except the intensity differs. For starters, you'll notice the program on the opposite page takes nearly a full hour for less than a half-dozen exercises per session. Granted, that's a lot of time, but that's what it generally takes because you're lifting extremely heavy weights and need to rest between sets. If you don't have that much time, concentrate on the exercises most important to you, say bench-pressing for your chest, shoulders and triceps or curling for heftier arms.

Here are other power-building strategies from fitness experts that differ from your standard workout. Keep them in mind before you start bulking up.

Take more time to recover. Muscles are like accountants after the federal income tax deadline: They need lots of R and R after working so hard.

"Recovery time is as important or maybe more important than the exercises themselves," says James E. Graves, Ph.D., associate professor and chair of the Department of Health and Education at Syracuse University in New York. For maximum rebuilding, he suggests 24 to 36 hours of rest between high intensity workouts.

One study at the University of South Carolina suggests you can gain muscle strength faster by resting a full 48 hours between workouts. Athletes there who did a five-set bench-press program rested either 24 or 48 hours between workouts. After 24 hours their performance declined 10 percent; after 48 hours they were able to equal or beat their maximum press.

Use a spotter. Proper technique is paramount if you want to avoid the possibility of injury, says Graham. Be smart and perfect your lifting technique before piling on extra plates. And always use a friend to spot you while you lift.

Make safe lifting a cinch. When performing overhead lifts or squats, cinch on a weight belt for added support to your lower back. "Infrequent use of a lifting belt can

---

Building Bigger Muscles

The following program was devised by Kent State University's Dr. Peter Lemon to help participants in his muscle studies gain mass. It's intended for guys who already are in good shape and want to reach the next level. If you follow this program and pay close attention to diet, you should see results in about six weeks. Remember, for each exercise, do six to ten reps per set, three sets total. The weight should be about 70 to 85 percent of the maximum you can lift one time.

Monday	Wednesday
Traditional squats	Bench presses
Leg presses	Incline presses
Leg extensions	Upright rows
Leg curls	Triceps extensions
Heel raises	

Friday	
Lat pull-downs	Bent-over rows
Seated pulley rows	Biceps curls

You'll notice this program works each muscle group only once a week. The legs are worked on Mondays, the chest on Wednesdays, the back on Fridays. That's because Dr. Lemon—and other researchers as well—believe muscles need maxing out only one day a week to get the most gains.

---

provide additional strengthening to the abdominal and lower back muscles," Graham says.

Pull on the gloves. Relax, you don't have to go the distance with George Foreman. We're talking about weight-lifting gloves. Gloves protect your hands from calluses, plus they give you a little extra gripping power, says Graham, which will help reduce the chance of injury from accidentally dropping a weight on your toes.

Endurance Programs

Power to Go the Distance

Your favorite football team is a steamrolling marvel—for the first three quarters. Then they get pounded so miserably in the fourth that they seem to have totally run out of, well, steam.

Which just might be the case. Conditioning experts say such a performance is typical of a team that has ignored endurance training. Most people think of football as a sport of slam-bang explosive strength. But when that kind of effort is called for repeatedly on the field, the game becomes a test of endurance. Endurance training, fitness experts say, is a wise tactic for just about any sport, whether it's played in bursts of strength as with football, at moderate intensity as with baseball or at a rhythmic cadence as with long-distance cycling.

"We need resistance training to maintain muscle tissue, but we also need aerobic enhancement to give us stamina," says Carlos DeJesus, a world-champion bodybuilder and fitness trainer in Richmond, Virginia. "I tell my clients, 'You're going to gain functional muscle tissue. It'll be the kind of muscle you need to play all day with the kids, or to haul in the groceries or to become involved in recreational sports—strength that you need.' I combine resistance training with aerobic conditioning to give them the best of both worlds."

Two Workouts in One

Athletic endurance has two components: muscular and cardiovascular. With muscular endurance the improvement shows up only in the muscle getting the exercise. Train your biceps for endurance, and you can lift babies or garbage cans all day long, but it won't make you a better runner. Cardiovascular endurance, however, is a whole-body phenomenon, an overall improvement in the ability of your heart, blood vessels and lungs to pump oxygen-rich blood to all parts of your body.

You can develop both kinds of endurance with a tactic called circuit training. Here's the general approach: Exercises are done in an established order, hitting the larger muscle groups first. To keep the heart rate up, use short rest periods between exercises—15 to 30 seconds. Do not hit the same muscles on two exercises in a row.

This nonstop method works both the muscles and the cardiovascular system. Sure, fitness experts say running, cycling and swimming are superior exercises for pure aerobic benefit. But the attractive thing about circuit training is its efficiency—you get two workouts at once.

To compare the cardiovascular benefits you get from running and weight lifting, researchers at Oregon Health Sciences University in Portland put 30 sedentary men through 16 weeks of training. One group ran three times a week for a minimum of 45 minutes per workout. A second group lifted weights three times a week for a minimum of 45 minutes. Over the 16 weeks both groups lost body fat and lowered their heart rate and blood pressure. Only the weight lifters increased muscle, and only the runners improved their oxygen uptake.

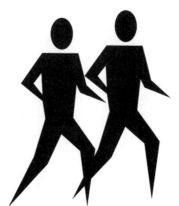

Get Specific

To tailor a training routine to your needs, consider what activity you're trying to perfect and what muscles are in-

volved. Most of us have an even mixture of fast- and slow-twitch muscle
fibers. The slow-twitch variety, which
burns oxygen for energy, is used in
long-and-steady endurance sports. You
get the most endurance gains in the
muscles you've targeted when you're
lifting light weights (ones that you can
lift for 20 to 30 repetitions). The most
brute-strength gains come with heavy
weights (ones you can lift for 4 to 6
repetitions). (The amount of weight
that you can lift for 8 to 12 repetitions
provides a mixture of strength and endurance.) So if you want to be a long-
distance swimmer, for example, you'll
want plenty of high-rep lifting for your
shoulders and arms, hips and knee
joints.

With this type of endurance
training, DeJesus says he's in condition
to run several miles even though he
doesn't hit the track regularly. His
lower back and ankles, he says, can't
take the trauma of regular jogging.
"But the way I train, I have the where-
withal—the lung capacity, aerobic
conditioning and strength—to run five
miles at any point," he says. "My legs
are strong, my lungs are strong. I don't
run five miles, but I'm conditioned to
be able to."

Aside from the aerobic aspects
of a workout, strength training benefits the heart in other ways. It can raise
concentrations of "good" cholesterol
(HDL) in the blood, for instance, and
can lower blood pressure in some
people with borderline high blood
pressure. It also can reduce the risk of
a heart attack caused by unaccustomed exertion. (The downside of that
is, of course, that you'll lose an excuse
for not shoveling snow off the sidewalk.)

Your Body: A History Lesson

View your body through a trainer's eyes. Fitness trainer Carlos DeJesus asks his clients the following questions before starting them on a circuit-training program. If the questions raise any red flags, be sure to talk to your doctor.

Health

• Have you ever had rheumatic fever, heart murmur, high blood pressure, heart attack, irregular heart rate, angina pectoris, abnormal electrocardiogram (EKG), artery disease, varicose veins, lung disease, epilepsy, diabetes or stroke?

• Have any of your family members, including parents and grandparents, had heart attacks before age 50, heart operations, high blood pressure, high cholesterol, diabetes or congenital heart disease?

• Have you had chest pain, shortness of breath, heart palpitations, lightheadedness, coughing on exertion, coughing up blood, back pain or joint stiffness?

Activity Level

Is your primary occupation sedentary? Do you walk less than one to two miles a day? Has your doctor ever told you you had high blood pressure? Has your doctor said or do you think you are 15 pounds or more overweight? Do you know your blood cholesterol level?

• When exercising, have you ever experienced shortness of breath, chest pain, joint discomfort or lower back pain?

General Questions

Would you say you're under moderate or extreme stress? Do you actively attempt to control your level of stress? Do you smoke, or have you in the past? Are you currently taking any medication? Anything else? (Consider factors such as back trouble, sprains, bone breaks, dislocations, recent surgery, kidney or circulation problems, allergies, asthma, hyperglycemia, hypoglycemia and the number of hours of sleep you get each day.)

Get Ready, Get Set . . .

First things first. When DeJesus's clients walk in the door, they go straight to the stationary bicycle for a five-minute warm-up. Then they do a series of stretches for 30 seconds each: hamstrings, quads, calves, back, chest, shoulders, biceps, triceps.

"You have to warm up," DeJesus says. "You hardly ever see a pitcher get out there cold and start pitching a ball at 100 miles an hour. He starts pitching from 15 feet away, 20 feet away, 25 feet away. And before you know it, he's pitching a rocket from the mound to home plate."

After the workout, cool down with light activity until your heart rate and breathing have returned to normal. Then repeat the same set of stretches.

What Makes Weight Lifting Aerobic?

You have every right to be baffled. Aerobics—isn't that dancing around to music? So how come people say weight lifting can be aerobic, too?

Aerobic exercise is any repetitive physical activity that improves the function of the heart, lungs and blood vessels. For pure aerobic conditioning, fitness experts say such activities as running, swimming and cycling are most effective. Weight lifting done with just 15 to 30 seconds of rest between exercises, however, also gives significant aerobic improvement and strengthens muscle at the same time. That makes it a particularly efficient form of conditioning.

These are the criteria that make an activity aerobic.

- It uses large muscle groups.
- You can keep it going for more than a

Working the Circuit

To build power that lasts all day, we turned to Carlos DeJesus, a world-champion bodybuilder and fitness trainer, who prescribes a combination of endurance and strength training. DeJesus suggests three weight-lifting sessions per week, with at least 48 hours between sessions to let your muscles recuperate.

The first and third sessions—done on Monday and Friday, for example—focus on muscular endurance: low weights for 20 to 25 reps. His aerobic circuit consists of four exercises: squats, lat pull-downs, deadlifts (if you have a bad back you can substitute back extensions or leg curls) and a bench press. Do them in the order listed and take two seconds for the "positive" phase and two seconds for the "negative" phase.

To keep the heart rate up, allow no more than 30 seconds between exercises. (University of Idaho researchers found 15 seconds to be optimal. At the very least, keep your rest interval shorter than your lifting period.) When you have completed the circuit, repeat it once or twice until you've been lifting for 35 to 40 minutes.

For the strength workout, which would be done on Wednesday if your other lifting days are Monday and Friday, he prescribes two series of exercises that should be alternated from one weekly session to the next. That

few minutes, raising the heart rate.
- It makes you perspire and breathe more heavily, without causing a "burn" in the muscles.

"We're going to be hearing more and more about using weights for aerobic activity," says DeJesus. "We're not just dancing. If that's all that you do, you risk losing muscle tissue. I have aerobics instructors who come to me because that's happened. They overuse their limbs way, you'll be less likely to get bored, and you'll hit a slightly different lineup of muscles. Stick to the order given. For balance, the exercises work muscles on one side of a joint and then the opposing muscles on the other side. Use a medium weight and perform 8 to 12 repetitions of each exercise. Take four seconds in the "positive" phase and two seconds for the "negative" phase. Do two or three sets.

These exercises are illustrated in part two of this book.

Strength Program A: Leg extensions (quads), leg curls (hamstrings), standing calf machine or heel raises, bench presses (chest), lat pull-downs (back), military presses (shoulders), barbell curls (biceps), triceps pull-downs and your choice of abdominal exercise.

Strength Program B: Squats (quads), stiff-legged deadlifts (lower back), seated calf machine or heel raises, dips (chest), bent-over rows (back), upright rows (shoulders), dumbbell curls (biceps) (grasp dumbbells as you would if you were doing a barbell curl, palm up, and raise both dumbbells at the same time), seated overhead extensions with narrow grip (triceps), shoulder shrugs (traps) and an abdominal exercise of your choice (for variety, choose a different exercise for program B).

for endurance, DeJesus suggests taking two seconds for the "positive" phase of the lift (the pushing up part of a bench press, for instance) and two seconds for the "negative" phase (lowering). So hire a band director for each of your workouts. Or, if you're on a budget, drop by a music store and pick up a beeping metronome to keep your lifting honest. Or you could make a tape of the metronome beat to help you keep your cadence.

Mind the store. If you're not working with a coach or a trainer, who's left to keep you accountable for the success of your workouts? Just you. So chart your progress at least once a week: Measure your waist, step on the scale and keep a chart of the weights and reps you use.

Get flexible. Stretching is not only for before and after lifting weights. Do your complete stretching routine before any recreational activity and even as a separate flexibility workout—say, the moment you roll out of bed. "People assume they can just bolt into a run from a cold muscle stage and everything's going to be okay," says DeJesus. "You've seen boxers warming up. You know why? Because they're going to get into the ring and throw a punch as hard as they can, and if you throw a punch as hard as you can, you can pull a muscle."

Treat yourself. If you've put yourself on a rigid eating plan, allow yourself an anything-goes meal once a week. "Don't be overly concerned if you stray from your meal plan," says DeJesus. "My wife and I eat 21 meals a week. For one of them, we eat whatever we want. And you know what that does? That ensures that we're going to stay on that other 20. It's a factored-in relief valve."

and they don't have enough conditioning to keep their muscle, so they have to do strength training once a week.

"When you weight-train, the body says, 'Uh-oh, you need this muscle tissue. You'd better go to another energy source. You have to use body fat as fuel for this activity.' "

Here's more advice for getting the most out of an endurance routine.

Keep time. When you're lifting weights

Flexibility Programs

Stretching Your Power

You're at a party. The conversation is flowing and so are the drinks. Suddenly, some joker suggests a game of limbo. Do you: (a) belly up to the limbo bar and glide under with the greatest of ease or (b) belly up to the real bar and see how far you can stretch a scotch-and-soda?

We're not saying flexibility will make you the life of the party, but it can provide physical and mental benefits that might surprise you. Whether you're a marathoner, bodybuilder or mountain climber, flexibility prevents injury, increases range of motion, promotes relaxation, reduces stress and keeps your body feeling loose and lubricated.

"You don't have to be Gumby, but it's important to maintain flexibility even if you're not a karate master," says John Skowron, a physical therapist at Raleigh Community Sports Medicine and Physical Therapy in Raleigh, North Carolina. "Flexibility gives you three-dimensional fitness. Without it, you're missing an important part of overall health."

Look Better, Feel Better

The range of motion for any joint is defined primarily by the elasticity of the muscles and tendons attached to it. So the point of stretching is to make your muscles loose and elastic so your joints can bend as smoothly and widely as possible. Ignore stretching, however, and you regress. Unused muscles become shorter and tighter over time, limiting your ability to move freely.

Let's banish a myth: There's no evidence that you lose flexibility as you gain muscle, providing you stretch as much as you lift. In fact, studies show your lifting can actually improve if your muscles are well-stretched.

"Stretching helps increase range of motion and should be a part of every general fitness program," says Steve J. Fleck, Ph.D., a sports physiologist in the Sports Science and Technology Division of the U.S. Olympic Committee in Colorado Springs, Colorado. "If you're already doing full range-of-motion resistance training, then research suggests that this muscle-building shouldn't have a negative impact on your flexibility."

Stretching is one of the few types of exercise you can safely do daily. It's also something you should do before and after every workout, adds Skowron. Warm up before stretching by doing five to ten minutes of jumping rope, jogging or light calisthenics to get the blood pumping. Then hold each stretch for 20 seconds or more. This overcomes your muscles' proclivity to contract when stretched, which is their defense against being stretched too far.

Stretch until you feel the tension in your muscles and hold it. Don't force yourself to go farther than you comfortably can, says Skowron, and don't bounce. That's ballistic stretching and it's as dangerous as it sounds.

"Stretching can help you everywhere in life, whether you're playing golf, basketball or racquetball," says fitness consultant and lecturer Laura A. Gladwin. "Even if you're a homebody, flexibility can help you perform activities of

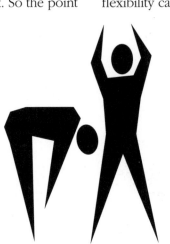

daily living such as shoveling snow or raking leaves."

If that's not motivation enough, Gladwin says, consider this: "Flexibility will boost your appearance by improving your posture and by slowing down the aging process by keeping you more mobile in your later years."

Here's how to embark on your own joint ventures of flexibility.

Neck
Head Turn

With your head in an upright position, simply turn to the left as far as you can and hold it for four to six seconds. Repeat on the right side. Gently rotate your head back to center in an upright position. Look down toward your chest and hold for four to six seconds; then return to starting position. Don't tilt your head back, lift your chin toward the ceiling or rotate your head in a circular motion. These movements place too much stress on the delicate vertebrae in your neck.

Shoulders
Shoulder Roll

From an upright position lift your shoulders up and in toward your chest. Then lower them down and out toward your back. Rotate them in a slow forward circular pattern through as much range of motion as possible; then repeat rotating in the opposite direction.

Shoulders, Upper Body
Overhead Shoulder Stretch

Stand erect, shoulders back, chest out, feet about shoulder-width apart. Raise your right arm overhead, with your elbow bent and your hand resting between your shoulder blades. Keep your left hand at your side.

Keeping your position, take your left hand and gently push on your right elbow, edging it to the center of your body and farther down behind your neck. Repeat, stretching the other arm.

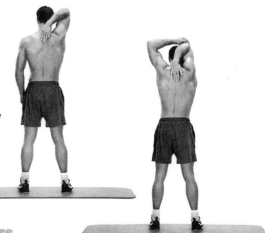

Chest and Shoulders
Chest Stretch

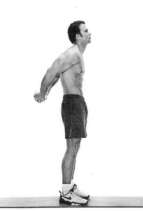

Stand erect with shoulders back, chest out and feet shoulder-width apart. Clasp your hands behind your back so your fingers are interlaced at about butt height. Now lift your arms in unison up and away from your body until you feel your chest and shoulder muscles stretching. Don't hunch over, and keep your chest out and chin in. Reach your hands for the ceiling, then lower.

Hips, Inner Groin
Hip Stretch

From a standing position take a large lunging step out with your right foot until your feet are a few feet apart. Lean into your right leg so your leg is bent at a 90-degree angle and your knee is directly over your ankle. Your rear leg is slightly bent and extended behind you. Put your hands on the floor for support. Now push your hip down and forward until you feel the stretch. Hold, repeat on the other leg.

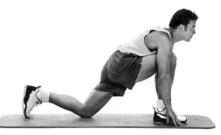

Back, Hips
Spinal Twist

Sit on the floor with both legs extended. Bend your right leg over your left leg, keeping your right foot flat on the floor outside the left knee. Place your left elbow on the outside of your right knee, and extend your right arm behind you with your palm flat on the floor for support.

Twist your upper body to the right by slowly looking over your right shoulder. Apply pressure with your left elbow on the outside of your right knee as you twist. Keep your upper body straight. Hold, switch sides, repeat.

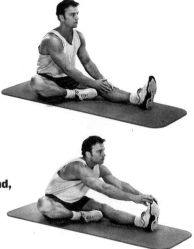

Calves
Calf Stretch

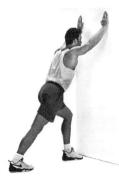

Stand a few feet away from a wall, feet about shoulder-width apart. Step forward with your left foot and bend your torso over at a slight angle so your hands are resting against the wall. Bend your left knee and extend your right leg behind you with the knee straight and heel flat. Keeping your back straight and toes forward, push your hips in toward the wall, feeling the stretch in your lower right leg and calf. Hold, repeat on the other leg.

Hamstrings, Lower Back, Hips
Hurdler's Stretch

Sit on the floor with both legs extended in front. Bring your right leg up and into your body, so that the sole of your right foot is against the inside thigh of your left leg, somewhere around the knee. Keep your left knee unlocked and slightly flexed, and your upper body upright, with back straight and arms in front.

Keeping your back straight, bend over at the hips and reach for the toes on your left foot. Pull your toes back slightly toward your upper body. Keep your legs on the ground, with your left knee unlocked. Switch legs, repeat.

Thighs
Quadriceps Stretch

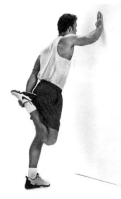

Stand a few inches away from a wall, with feet shoulder-width apart. Place your right hand against the wall for balance, and bend your right knee, raising your right foot behind your body until you can grasp it with your left hand. Keep your thigh perpendicular to the floor, and gently pull your heel in toward your butt until you feel a stretch in your right thigh. Repeat on the other leg.

The ⌂ **next** level

Note: **These splits are for advanced stretchers only. If you can't do them properly, go as far as you comfortably can, hold, then relax and repeat. Take it easy—they'll take time and effort to perfect.**

Groin, Hamstrings, Hips: **Forward Split**

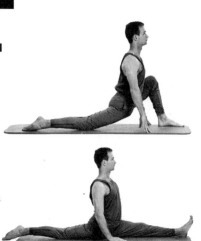

Stand upright, feet hip-width apart, with your left foot behind you as if you had just taken a big step backward. Lean into your right leg, which should be bent at about a 90-degree angle with your foot firmly on the floor. Your left foot should be top-down on the floor, sliding out and back behind you.

Slide your left foot back and your right foot forward as far as you can go, until your hips sink to the floor in a fully forward front split. Your upper body should be upright with a slight forward lean to it.

Groin, Hamstrings, Hips: **Side Split**

From a standing position take a large step to the side with your left leg. Keep both feet in line with each other, with your toes slightly pointed out away from your body. Bend over at the waist with your hands on the ground for support, and spread your legs as far apart as you can, but not fully in split position.

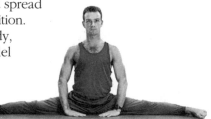

Slowly slide your feet out to the sides of your body, sinking your hips to the floor. Your legs should be parallel to the floor, with your groin against the floor. Use your hands in front for support.

Back, Stomach, Upper Body:
Cobra Stretch

Lie on your stomach with your palms flat on the ground at your sides, halfway between your hips and shoulders. Keep your legs together, with feet on their tops, toes pointing away from your body. Elbows should be bent at a 90-degree angle and eyes forward.

Keeping your legs together, lift your upper body up off the ground, inhaling as you rise. Press your hips into the floor, and curve your upper body backward, looking up. Puff your chest out and pull back your shoulders. (Hands may be slid forward slightly for more support if you need it.) Your body should look like a cobra ready to strike. Breathe regularly while in position, then exhale as you lower yourself.

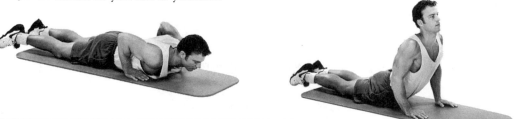

Quest for the Best

They're world-beaters: successful, celebrated and at the top of their games. Being the best is more than just a goal for these guys. It's a way of life. Here are their secrets for staying powerfully fit.

Tommy Moe, Olympic Ski Champ

King of the Downhill

Ask the pundits: Not one of them expected great things—or *any*thing—from the U.S. Alpine Ski Team heading into the 1994 Winter Olympics in Lillehammer, Norway. *Sports Illustrated*, in its Winter Olympic preview issue, dismissed them as "woeful," dubbing the team a "lead-footed snowplow brigade."

Tommy Moe, who had placed a disappointing 20th in the men's downhill at the 1992 Olympics, was determined to prove the critics wrong. "It bugged me a little, because I really didn't think we deserved it," the Alaskan, who is in his mid-twenties, recalls. And prove them wrong he did.

At Lillehammer, in five-degree weather, in front of 30,000 stunned spectators, Moe rocketed down the icy track on a flawless run that earned him the gold medal in men's downhill. In doing so, he led a charge that earned the U.S. ski team five medals in the first ten days of the Olympics— including another medal for Moe, who took the silver in the Super G competition.

Two weeks after slamming the ski team, *Sports Illustrated* ate its words, featuring Tommy on the cover. And a proud American public was calling for Moe.

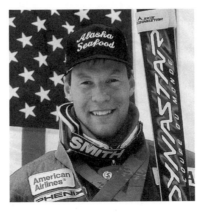

Building Moe-mentum

Moe owes his success to an absolute knowledge of his abilities. His coaches have marveled at the speeds he can handle— upwards of 90 miles an hour—and his razor-sharp precision executing turns at that velocity. But Moe is the first to admit he wouldn't have the control—or the ability—without an eclectic fitness regimen that keeps mind and body honed as sharp as a ski's edge.

"When I'm training for the winter, I try to follow a six-day program. Monday, Wednesday and Friday are my weight-training days. On Tuesday, Thursday and Saturday, though, I mix it up with some other sports to get a good aerobic workout," he says. For Moe that could mean anything from hiking to kayaking.

Although he advocates as much of a total-body workout as possible, Moe devotes most of his weight training to his legs, abdominals and lower back. "They're the foundation. People think it's just the legs, but you use your back and torso a lot—it's where your center of balance is." So Moe strengthens that center with plenty of crunches, sidebends and leg lifts.

Then he subjects his legs to a battery of grueling exercises: leg curls, squats, tuck jumps and box jumps—where Moe literally jumps on and off a foot-high box as many times as he can in a minute. "The jump exercises are great for the leg strength you need when you have to change position quickly on a run," he says.

When he's not competing, Moe has little trouble staying in skiing shape. "I just try to do a lot of activities that require the same skills I use in skiing—balance and reaction time, especially." Moe's favorites include kayaking and mountain biking. "The kayak fine-tunes your balance because you always have to be careful not to tip over. And in either sport you always have to be looking ahead, reading the terrain, because stuff is flashing by really quickly," he says. But Moe's most important off-season workout is the minimum three hours a week he spends on in-line skates. "It's about the closest thing to skiing—it really helps me keep in form."

Fuel to Burn

Moe's five-foot-ten, 200-pound body is ideal for skiing, and he helps keep it that way with a surprisingly average diet most of us would be glad to follow.

"Basically, I eat whatever I want. For breakfast I'll have cereal, bread, bagels, pancakes, even eggs. I eat lots of fruit. For dinner I love pasta or steak," he says. "When I'm in Alaska, I'll eat tons of salmon and halibut. And I gotta say, I like drinking a beer after a hard day of skiing—it tastes pretty damn good."

But don't be misled by his omnivorous attitude. "As a skier, I need a lot of calories. It helps keep an extra layer of insulation on me so the cold won't interfere with my performance," he says. And although Moe eats what he wants, he still watches out for the saturated fats that could clog up his high-performance heart. "I'm not big on butter. I don't eat a lot of bacon or mayonnaise. And yeah, I'll have a steak, but I make sure it's a good lean cut, and I cut the excess fat off," he says. Even with his

How He Does It

Monday/Wednesday/Friday

Lunges	3 sets, 8 reps
Squats	3 sets, 8 reps
Leg extensions	3 sets, 8 reps
Leg curls	3 sets, 8 reps
Calf raises	3 sets, 8 reps
Strutting (walking on heels, toes elevated)	3–5 minutes
Crunches	2 sets, 20 reps
Leg raises	2 sets, 20 reps
Sidebends	2 sets, 20 reps
Seated leg tucks	2 sets, 20 reps
Tuck jumps	1 minute
Box jumps	1 minute

Tuesday/Thursday/Saturday

Stretching	A few minutes
Running	1 mile
Sprints	400 yards, 3 times 200 yards, 4 times
Outdoor activities (In-line skating, speed-hiking, mountain biking or kayaking)	1 hour

"extra layer of insulation," Moe's body fat is just 8 percent.

Although Moe might allow himself a few dietary excesses, when it comes to his overall fitness regimen, he doesn't cut himself any slack. "If you want to get anywhere, you always have to push yourself as hard as you can," he says. "Whether you're doing a rep or a set, or taking a hill on skis or a mountain bike, you have to push it, you have to challenge yourself. Try to do a little bit more than you think you can. Don't give up. Keep pushing, keep digging."

Marty Nothstein, World-Champion Cyclist

Powering His Way to Gold

Lying awake at night, his heel throbbing with pain, Marty Nothstein was sure his cycling season—and his dreams of gold—were over. Just three weeks before the 1994 national championships, he had fractured his heel bone in a crash. Nothstein had worked hard through the harshest winter in memory to get himself in the best shape of his life—gold medal shape—and now he couldn't even walk. His doctors told him he would be in a cast for two months— the time remaining before the world championships.

"After many sleepless nights, I said I worked way too hard this winter to let it all slip through my hands," Nothstein, who is in his mid-twenties, recalls. "I told the doctor, 'I'm taking a chance. I want to ride. I want to race.'"

Still unable to walk, Nothstein discarded his cast and returned to the gym, working on leg machines and doing upper-body exercises. He kept up his aerobic capacity by swimming against strong currents generated by a training flume at the nearby Allentown Sports Medicine and Human Performance Center. "After rehab my foot would hurt so bad I'd actually just sit at home and cry," he says. "The memory of that helped a lot mentally when I was racing. I thought, 'All that pain I've been through—I deserve to win.'"

In a real-life tale of courage and perseverance that makes *Rocky* seem like a PBS documentary, Nothstein won the keirin—a frenetic 1666.5 meter race in which cyclists jockey for position behind a pacesetting motorcycle for 3½ laps and then unleash a furious lap-and-a-half sprint to the finish—and took second in the match sprint at the national

championships. And just two months after fracturing his heel bone, he became the first American man in 82 years to win a gold medal in the world championships match sprint. But Nothstein was just getting warmed up. He then rode to gold in the keirin, becoming the first American man ever to win two gold medals at the Worlds.

"One reason I came back so quickly is my big base of power training and all my endurance training on the road," Nothstein says. "My body had something to feed off of when it was injured."

Pedaling Power

The explosive power Nothstein brings to his sport begins in the gym. "I emphasize weight training pretty much all through the year," Nothstein says.

Lean and sinewy at six feet two inches and 210 pounds, Nothstein brings the same ferocious intensity to the gym that he uses to blow competitors off the track. During his power-training phase he does squats with up to 450 pounds, cleans with 225 pounds and dead-lifts with up to 350 pounds. He has leg-pressed more than 1,100 pounds.

All of Nothstein's weight training, however, is designed to build power specifically for cycling. "I know tons of guys who can lift a lot more weight than me," Nothstein says. "But it all comes down to transmitting it on the bicycle—who can push the pedals harder and faster."

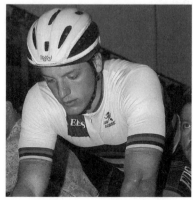

Training Wheels

Marty Nothstein grew up a stone's throw from the Lehigh County Velodrome in Trexlertown, Pennsylvania.

Literally.

If it hadn't been for a stone-throwing contest with his

younger brother, Jason, Nothstein might never have become a world champion.

"We were bored," Nothstein says, with an impish grin. "So we were throwing rocks, to see how far we could throw them. And before you know it, we hit this guy's house a few times."

The guy who owned the house turned out to be Heinz Walter, a former cycling coach. When Nothstein's mother made the two teenagers go over to apologize to Walter, he suggested they join the developmental cycling program at the nearby velodrome.

"He said, 'I see you kids on your bikes all the time. Try it.' And that's how I got introduced to cycling," Nothstein recalls.

Nothstein entered the local racing scene when he was 16, and over the next four years rose to national class largely on the basis of his natural talent. But after finishing a disappointing seventh in the 1991 Pan Am Games, Nothstein realized he needed to devote himself entirely to his sport if he wanted to take the next step up to world-class level.

By 1993 he had a world championship silver medal in the keirin to show for his dedication, followed by his incredible gold medal double in 1994. In 1995 Nothstein made a triumphant return to the Pan Am Games, powering his way to a gold medal in the match sprint and setting a Pan Am Games record in the process.

"I'm still at that training point where if I train hard, I'm going to reap the benefits. And the benefits are great. I'm living a dream."

Nothstein knows what it takes to be a champion. And the same rules apply whether you're on the fast track at a corporation or a velodrome, he says. "Even in life, if you want to

be the best CEO of a company, you're going to have to really put your head to it and go at it harder than anyone else does," Nothstein says. "It relates into sports also. The hard trainers are the guys who are making it to the top."

"The goal, of course, is winning—winning some more world titles along the way. It's become an obsession of mine," Nothstein says. "I know what hard work does. Hard work pays off. Whatever people say, the bottom line is hard work pays off."

How He Does It

To prepare for the summer cycling season, world champ Marty Nothstein goes into an intense power phase for weight training between March 1 and April 30. The following is his workout schedule in the gym. The Day One program is usually done Monday and Thursday; Day Two, on Tuesday and Friday. Nothstein usually warms up for most exercises by doing a set of ten reps with light weight, followed by a set of eight reps with slightly more weight. Then he goes into his routine with heavy weights.

Day One

Power cleans	3 sets, 5 reps
Dumbbell rows	3 sets, 6 reps
Dumbbell lunges	3 sets, 6 reps
Posterior raises	3 sets, 8 reps
Back extensions	3 sets, 20 reps

Day Two

Stiff-legged deadlifts	3 sets, 5 reps
Squats	3 sets, 6 reps
Bench presses with barbell	3 sets, 5 reps
Leg curls	3 sets, 6 reps
Crunches	3 sets, 20 reps
Crunches, with legs straight	3 sets, 20 reps
Crunches	3 sets, 20 reps
Crossover crunches	3 sets, 20 reps

Bob Arnot, M.D., CBS News Medical Correspondent

Keeping an Eye on Fitness

As a medical correspondent for CBS News since 1985, Dr. Bob Arnot is constantly on the go. In his late forties, he's never really been out of shape. A two-time Ironman Triathlon competitor and participant in over 100 triathlons, Dr. Arnot spent part of his career as the team physician for the U.S. Ski Team, and kept plenty fit on the slopes.

But like a lot of men, Dr. Arnot reached a point where he figured the onset of middle age and the demands of a fast-paced career were conspiring against him—and he'd have to say farewell to his former fit self.

A news assignment in Africa in 1994 changed that. "I was doing a story for CBS," he recalls. His assignment exposed him to the twin perils of cholera and dysentery. "When I came back from that extended trip, I was feeling even older than my age." That's when he said, "Physician, heal thyself!"

And he did. Dr. Arnot began interviewing medical and exercise experts from all disciplines, trying to devise the best possible health and fitness regimen for himself. He ended up writing his findings in the book *Dr. Bob Arnot's Guide to Turning Back the Clock.* In the process Dr. Arnot also transformed his six-foot-four frame into a trim, 200-pound paragon of fitness, with 7 percent body fat and 14 pounds of new muscle.

Today when he competes in his favorite sports, Dr. Arnot leaves guys half his age in his dust. "And I did it by taking charge of my health, my fitness, by not listening to those old paradigms," he says.

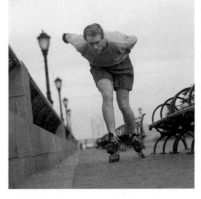

Instead, he began eating better and came to appreciate the need for a powerful workout routine. "My friends and I were lifelong aerobic animals. We always disdained bodybuilding—and that was a big mistake. I tell people now, if there's a fountain of youth, it's the heavy metal in your local gym," he says.

Fueling His Workouts

Dr. Arnot's workout begins early—with his commute to work in New York City. "I live in East Harlem, about four miles from the office. I'll either ride my bike there or use in-line skates. I do it every day, even in the winter. I keep a rack of clothes in my office and I change there."

Every day, Monday through Friday, Dr. Arnot hits the gym. He starts with an hour on the Alpine Trainer, a beast of a machine that looks like a stair-climber on steroids. "The steps are three times as long as your average climber. It also has plenty of bars on it where I can lay my papers and medical journals and work while I'm working out," he says. Then he spends about 40 minutes cycling and at least 40 minutes lifting weights. "I favor a weight-training regimen where you work a different group of muscles each day of the week. On Monday, for instance, you focus on just back exercises. Tuesday, maybe it's shoulders and abs. That way, you have a good variety to your workout and you'll never be too sore."

Dr. Arnot doesn't let an assignment get in the way of a workout, either. "When I'm on the road, I'll take my bike and my skates and tour the cities I'm in. I also try to stay in hotels that have exercise rooms or a fitness club nearby."

Exercise, however, is only half the answer, Dr. Arnot believes. "Being powerfully fit is as much about eating the right foods as it is about pumping weights," he says. "The more men learn to fuel for their workouts, the more powerful they'll be."

Dr. Arnot favors a diet heavy on slow-burning carbohydrates—foods such as high-fiber cereals, fruits and whole grains—and proteins—including yogurt, skim milk and lean meat. "Proteins build muscle. Slow-burning carbs keep your blood-sugar steady, so you won't crash during a workout," he says. And after a stint in the gym, Dr. Arnot immediately tops off the tank with a protein-filled sports beverage. "This is a controversial area, but it's had tremendous results for me."

Most men would probably have serious qualms about Dr. Arnot's self-imposed restrictions—his diet is extremely low in fat, with no red meat or alcohol. "But my nutrition allows me to do what I want, when I want—and with the energy of a 19-year-old," he says.

Forever Young

For the older guy who wants to get in shape, Dr. Arnot says it's never too late. But the earlier you start training, the longer you'll enjoy the benefits.

"Don't let yourself be programmed into believing you can't beat the kids at their own game. If you're willing, you can have the heart, lungs and body of a man 20 years younger than the date on your birth certificate." A big part of that, he says, is attitude. Dr. Arnot is living proof, actively competing in sports that most 47-year-old guys wouldn't even think of trying. "It's all part of being in better shape physically and mentally—don't be afraid to try new things," he says.

And don't be afraid to use your head, either. "A lot of young guys out there don't pace themselves, don't take their time to learn the proper technique of a sport or exercise—and don't have the buying power to afford the best training and equipment money can buy." Older athletes have three advantages, says Dr. Arnot: wisdom, experience and a bigger wallet. "Use them," he says.

How He Does It

Bob Arnot does four sets with 8 to 12 reps of the following excercises.

Monday

Pull-ups	Incline rows
Horizontal rows	Upright rows

Tuesday

Military presses	Deltoid machine
Vertical rows	Shrugs
Abdominal machine	Lower-ab crunches
Rotary twists	

Wednesday

Bench presses	Incline presses
Flies	Cable rows
Tricep presses	Leg presses
Lunges	

Thursday

Biceps curls	Preacher curls
Cable curls	Abdominal machine
Lower-ab crunches	Rotary twists

Friday

Triceps dips	Triceps pull-downs
Triceps inverted preachers	Leg presses
Lunges	

Saturday/Sunday (any of the following)

Cross-country skiing	Mountain biking
Kayaking	Tennis
Alpine skiing	

Joe Lewis, Former World Karate Champion

Putting the Power in Empowerment

Joe Lewis is the Muhammad Ali of karate fighting: simply The Greatest. He learned karate while serving in the Marines, earned a tenth-degree black belt and trained with Bruce Lee. In his fighting career he garnered more titles than a small library and was voted "The Greatest Karate Fighter of All Time."

But Lewis doesn't preach a dogma of discipline when it comes to exercise. Now in his early fifties, he's as much a philosopher as he is a fighter. And his words of wisdom pack as much power as his jabs and kicks.

"I don't go over all the health reasons for working out. You hear that junk every day from medical experts and so-called experts," Lewis says in his light North Carolina accent. "For me exercise is trying to balance out the phenomena of hard work and having fun, follow me?

"Too often guys go to the gym and it becomes a duty. Anything that's a duty, you tend to become irresponsible with, and that's no way to motivate yourself," he says. "People used to think I was rude because I didn't talk to anybody in the gym. I came in, worked out and left. That was okay for me, but for most other people, working out should be fun."

From Farm Boy to World Champ

Lewis grew up with four brothers. His father was a full-time college professor who still worked the family farm every day. Lewis's father preferred an old-fashioned way of life: He plowed the soil by hand instead of using a tractor, and when he got sick (which he rarely did),

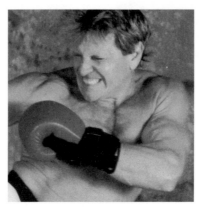

he relied on home remedies and avoided doctors.

"If he were about to come down with a cold, he'd buy a bag of oranges and sit down and eat nearly every one of them," Lewis says.

At 14, Lewis began weight lifting with the same dedication and zeal he'd later apply to karate. "I always thought that a muscular body was a beautiful body. It has an aesthetic appeal. It has power," Lewis says. "Even as a boy, that look appealed to me. I'd run to the store just to pick up the muscle magazines."

By 19, Lewis beefed up to 225 pounds. He also joined the service. After a few weeks of seasickness en route to Okinawa, he dropped ten pounds and took up martial arts training under three native instructors.

"Around that time I got turned off to weight lifting a little bit because I started getting stretch marks on my thighs and chest," he says. "They kept getting bigger and bigger, and I didn't like that. I thought they were disgusting. It's not necessary to blow your body up like a balloon."

Lewis eventually received his black belt in Shorinryu karate, a Japanese martial art. He gained an enviable reputation for his prowess by teaching fellow servicemen hand-to-hand combat in Vietnam. In 1966, at age 24, he became the amateur world karate champion in the point-fighting system. By 1971 he migrated to kickboxing and became the U.S. heavyweight champ. (Kickboxers fight continuously with full-contact blows, much like boxing; point-fighters fight with controlled blows to score points by hitting specific body parts.)

Before long Lewis was making action movies, co-hosting a talk show on martial arts and appearing in the popular media. His career culminated in 1983, when he was voted "Greatest Karate Fighter of All Time" in a *Karate*

Illustrated survey. Nine years earlier, he had a similar honor bestowed on him by the French publication *Karate*.

Fighting the Good Fight

Lewis doesn't fight competitively anymore. But he still appears at karate functions around the country. He also makes training videotapes. He's produced over 20 of them on everything from fighting technique to weight lifting for martial artists. Like him, they're folksy and no-frills, but packed with wisdom he's acquired through the decades.

Lewis's biggest project these days is giving self-defense seminars, especially to senior citizens. He won two North Carolina governor's awards for his educational efforts in crime prevention.

When he's not on the road, Lewis works out several days a week by mixing weight lifting and martial arts. "I mix it up a lot. You have to. That's part of making it fun," he says.

As for diet, Lewis sticks to what he likes best, tempered with common sense. "I'm turned off by the traditional American breakfast of eggs and bacon. I've conditioned myself to like foods that are good for me. I try to eat a salad with my meats, and I eat red meat only once a week or so. I also eat my food plain—no garnish, butter or salt."

Lewis's only quirk is that he eats his dessert first and salad last. "It started when I was a kid," he says.

But whether he's eating lunch or throwing a punch, Lewis's message of empowerment shines through everything he does. "My motivation comes through a personal feeling of responsibility. A feeling of personal empowerment. Weight lifting and martial arts can give you this confidence, too," he says. "But the most important thing to remember is that it's better to do some workout some of the time, than to do nothing all the time. If you can balance the hard work by having fun, you're going to stick with it."

How He Does It

Note: Joe Lewis mixes up his training regimen to keep things fun, plus he never forces a workout. "I let my body have a say-so in my daily schedule, so my workouts vary. I just listen to my body," he says.

Here's a typical week's workout.

Weight-lifting routine (once a week)

Upright rows	2 sets, 10 reps
Lat pull-downs	2 sets, 15 reps
Incline bench presses	2 sets, 10 reps
Bench presses	2 sets, 10 reps
Dumbbell flies	2 sets, 30 reps
Leg extensions	2 sets, 15 reps to failure
Leg curls	2 sets, 15 reps
Sit-ups with a twist	2 sets, 20–30 reps
Leg raises	2 sets, 30–50 reps
Stretching	15–20 minutes

Martial arts routine (several times a week)

Stretching	15 minutes
Heavy bag	4 to 5 3-minute rounds (punching)
	4 to 5 3-minute rounds (kicking)
Double-end bag (7-inch size)	3 to 4 3-minute rounds
Shadowboxing	15–20 minutes
Defense shadowboxing	1 to 2 3-minute rounds
Stretching (total body)	15–20 minutes

Michael Chang, Tennis Ace

Power Serves Star Well

When Michael Chang makes short work of an opponent on the tennis court, it's partly because of the long hours he spends working out in the gym.

Chang lifts weights up to two hours, three times a week, working on the muscles most critical to tennis.

"Weight training gave me a more powerful serve," Chang says. "In the pros everybody has a big serve. Everybody's acing each other ten times a match. If you're weak, you have to strengthen and try to turn your serve into an asset. Make it a weapon, so it can help you end your game and save you a lot of energy."

To improve his volleys, Chang builds his forearms with wrist curls and by squeezing a tennis ball. To add pop to his serve, he strengthens his shoulders with military presses and bent-over flies. To put more power behind *all* of his shots, Chang exercises his mid-section with crunches, seated barbell twists and dumbbell sidebends. "Weight transfer plays a part in generating power, which is why the mid-section is so important," Chang says. "It helps you get more power behind the ball."

To work his obliques (the muscles that run down the sides of the stomach and turn the torso), Chang plays catch with a trainer using a 15-pound medicine ball and rotating just his upper body. "All shots require twisting," says Chang, "so I do more abdominal work than anything else."

In 1989, at age 17, he became the youngest man ever to snare the French Open title. On the court his preparation, speed and guile have helped him reel in bigger, stronger opponents.

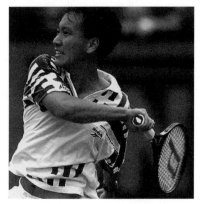

His training plan turned one of the smallest players on the men's tour into one of the most feared.

The year he burst onto the world scene, in 1989, Chang fractured his hip. The diagnosis: too much pounding aggravated by weak, inflexible hip muscles. Since then, he's become a devout stretcher. He keeps his back, buttocks and hamstrings limber, but the primary focus is on his hips.

His exercise of choice is admittedly bizarre, but it gets the job done: He gets down on all fours and rotates his hips in a circular motion—to the right side, back, to the left, then forward—for a few minutes at a time. "I'm probably the only guy who does this exercise, because it looks so weird," he says. "But I do more running than just about anyone else on the tour, so I need more flexibility in my hips."

Different Strokes

Chang has climbed to the top of the tennis rankings the old-fashioned way: through hard work and perseverence. There is no one secret to improving your game, he says.

"It's tricky. It varies," Chang says. "Take serving, for example. Goren Ivanisevic has a deceptive and effective serve. Great timing, but he tosses the ball low and serves on the rise. Pete Sampras doesn't snap his serve, but he's fluid with a good rhythm, gets the ball high and out in front. Other guys aren't real accurate, but have a lot of power. And then there's John McEnroe, who didn't serve hard, but placed his shots so well you weren't able to get them back. And if you did, it would just be an easy put-away for him.

"It's really a matter of what works for you, and practicing it enough to get yourself into a rhythm. Then add strength so you can add some pop to your serve. You can loosen the tension on your racquet to give you more power on your serve. You can try to get more spin, for control and accuracy."

Gone Fishing

Endurance, concentration, patience, stealth. Michael Chang brings these traits to his favorite sport: fishing.

"It takes so much preparation and technique to fish," he says. "First you decide what to fish for; then it's what type of boat; the hook; whether to use plastic worms, spinners, flies or live bait like wigglers, crayfish, lizards, mealworms or water dogs. It's such a big challenge."

Never Give Up

It's generally accepted in the tennis world that facing Chang is a losing proposition one way or the other. Even if you beat him, you'll be left with little energy to play the next match. Chang never gives up games or sets to conserve energy. He empties his tank every time. It's a strategy that pays a psychological dividend. "When you're out there, never stopping, that can be enough to beat someone," he says.

During play, which sometimes goes on for hours, he concentrates on each point and nothing else. He knows from experience that if he waits long enough, his opponent—Pete Sampras, Andre Agassi, the fish, it doesn't matter—might drop his guard and mess up. Says Chang: "Points turn into games. Games into sets. Sets into matches. Matches into tournaments. Tournaments into becoming number one."

Chang is a tireless scrambler who uses his speed to nullify the hard servers of the game. Part of his swiftness comes from his low center of gravity (he's five feet nine), but being speedy requires work. Each day, during two-

How He Does It

When he's in serious training, Michael Chang supplements his court time with weights and occasional running and swimming.

To stave off boredom, Chang varies his training schedule. In general, he spends four hours a day on the tennis court—two hours in the morning and two in the afternoon. He lifts weights up to two hours three days a week, focusing on the muscles crucial to tennis: shoulders, obliques (for twisting the mid-section), abdominals, back and forearms. He runs or does footwork drills two days a week.

hour morning and afternoon practices, Chang does precision footwork drills with his brother-turned-coach, Carl. First he does a series of sideways sprints, moving back and forth across the court as many as 20 times, keeping low and on his toes. Next he runs backward and forward from the net to the baseline. "I try to be really efficient with my movements," he says.

To keep his reflexes sharp, Chang has two trainers at the net fire tennis balls at him as he stands at the baseline, a mere 13 yards away, and works to return them. "They'll take turns and hit them high, low and all over the place," he says. Thirty minutes is about all he can take.

Chang admits to having a weak spot for cheeseburgers, pizza and most of the menu at Taco Bell, but his resolve hardens two weeks before a tournament. "No red meat, nothing fried or greasy and only an occasional dairy product," he says.

The mainstays: pasta, rice, tofu and Chinese food—"chicken and vegetables, very little oil, hold the MSG." He doesn't snack much, preferring instead to eat four big meals a day.

"I eat 1½ times what a normal person eats," Chang says. "When I'm in a restaurant, people look at me strange because I'm such a small person (145 pounds) eating so much."

Jim Howley, AIDS Activist and Triathlete

In the Race of His Life

Jim Howley is the type of guy who could make the rest of us green with envy. With his wavy blond hair, Southern California good looks and rippling muscles, Howley has always appeared in the peak of physical fitness. And the disgusting thing was, he didn't even have to work at it.

"Oh, I just have the kind of body that keeps muscle," he says with an almost infuriating nonchalance. "I really didn't need to think that much about fitness."

At least, not until 1983, when Howley tested positive for HIV—the virus that causes AIDS. "That really sent me into a tailspin. Even then, I didn't do anything good for my health—just the opposite in fact," he says. It wasn't until 1989, when he was diagnosed with full-blown AIDS, that Howley finally accepted his own mortality. Like most people faced with the impending threat of death, he experienced the classic fight-or-flight impulse. In the end Howley decided to run for his life.

"I just wanted to do something impossible. At the time the idea of running a marathon or triathlon seemed to fit the bill," he recalls.

So the morning after his AIDS diagnosis, Howley set out from his home near Santa Barbara, planning to run a mile. "A half-mile later, I was exhausted and had to crawl home. And I had been running downhill," he says.

A Reason to Run

But Howley kept at it. Within eight months he had completed his first marathon *and* his first triathlon. Since then, the course of his health has been dotted with obstacles—including a bout with testicular cancer—but they haven't slowed him down. When he's not running the hills near his home, Howley runs his own nonprofit organization, Athletics Instead of Depression and Sickness, which he founded in January 1994.

"It's my way of trying to promote physical activity as a weapon against AIDS," says Howley, who is in his mid-thirties. He counsels other AIDS patients and lectures at colleges around the country on the benefits of exercise. Working with the Physicians Association for AIDS Care, Howley even produced a personal exercise video for AIDS patients. "It was important for me to pass on that information. Let's face it: I should have died years ago, and exercise saved me."

Every year since his AIDS diagnosis, Howley has competed in the grueling Los Angeles Marathon—and every year, he's improved his time. In 1995 he ran a 4:10.

"The marathon was part of a deal I made with myself. When you have AIDS, it's very easy to make the disease your life. But if you do that, pretty soon you'll die. I decided to make athletics my life—and it's a choice that has allowed me to live."

The validity of Howley's decision is based as much in science as it is in attitude. "There's solid reasoning for exercise in AIDS treatment," says Howley. "When I got my diagnosis, I began studying up on things like physiology and saw the link. At first, doctors didn't want AIDS

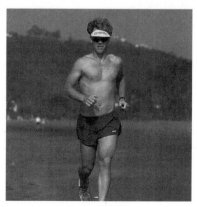

patients to exercise, but now they're recommending it."

The reason: lean muscle mass. Over 70 percent of lean muscle mass is needed to sustain life. "It's a key to resisting the ravages of the disease. If a person loses his lean muscle mass, the body doesn't have anything to work with to help fight off the disease." The need for life-sustaining muscle mass provides all the motivation Howley needs to keep working and competing.

But one gap in his athletic routine—and Howley shamefacedly admits it—is a consistent weight-training program. "I used to lift weights, but I found that bulking up really inhibited my form in sports like swimming." That said, Howley still enjoys the power workout of a triathlete, burning about 5,000 calories a day. During the weeks leading up to a triathlon, he runs about 50 miles, cycles around 150 miles and swims 3200 meters every night with a masters' group at his local pool. His road work doesn't pull any punches, either. "Whether I'm running or cycling, I'm always searching out hills, which are hard for me because of my size," says the six-foot, 192-pound Howley. "But they're great for building leg strength—hams, glutes, quads, you name it."

Balancing His Diet

Even more than most triathletes, Howley has to pay close attention to what he eats. "My system's pretty precarious," he says. "I can't digest things like I used to. Frankly, if a dish is prepared improperly, it could kill me. As you can imagine, I cook a lot of my own food."

High on his must-eat list are high-carbohydrate pastas and vegetables. Fats are at the bottom. "My system can't really break down a lot of fats anymore, but I need the calories. I used to be really fat-phobic, but I started dropping the pounds pretty fast. That was dangerous for me because of the disease. Plus, I didn't feel good in competition; when I finished a run, I'd be feverish." So now Howley has his fats in moderation: a little butter here, a little mayo there. "And if I feel up to it, I might

even have a nice, lean piece of filet mignon."

Having conquered the triathlon and the marathon, Howley still is looking for new heights to scale. One of his goals is to compete in the grueling Ironman triathlon at Kona, Hawaii. "I don't care what it takes—I'm going," he says. After that he'd like to get into a 50- or 100-mile ultramarathon run. "I like facing an ultimate challenge," he says. "Believe me, that's one thing AIDS prepares you for."

How He Does It

The following is Jim Howley's average training schedule.

Monday

Cycling (hilly terrain)	30–40 miles
Swimming	3200 meters

Tuesday

Running	6–8 miles
Stair-climbing	1 hour
Swimming	3200 meters

Wednesday

Cycling	60–70 miles
Swimming	500 meter sets

Thursday

Cycling	10 miles
Running (immediately after cycling)	3–4 miles
Swimming	3200 meters

Friday

Cycling	40–50 miles
Running	6–8 miles
Swimming	3200 meters

Saturday

Cycling	No set time limit
Tennis	No set time limit
In-line skating	No set time limit

Ashrita Furman, Guinness Record Holder

Tapping an Inner Power

Imagine Horatio Alger in a manic and surreal mood, bored silly with common success stories. He could easily have taken pen in hand and invented Ashrita Furman.

As a child, you see, Furman was not interested in anything athletic. Unless you count the pogo stick. And darn if Furman didn't grow up to be one of the world's most prominent pogo-stickers, ka-chunking his way through the piranha-infested waters of the Amazon River and up and down 16 miles of Mount Fuji's foothills, breaking world records all the way.

This isn't whimsical fiction. Furman, the fortysomething manager of a health food store in Jamaica, New York, has made a career of gathering number one citations in the Guinness Book of World Records. At any one time, his name can usually be found next to 10 or 11 titles for such pursuits as pogo-sticking, backwards unicycling, somersaulting, basketball dribbling, deep knee-bends and walking with a full milk bottle on his head.

Furman has broken Guinness records more than 40 times. While he has broken some records several times over, there's one event he will not be revisiting: underwater pogo-sticking.

"That was in the book for a couple of years, but they took it out," says Furman. "They said it was too dangerous. I pogo-sticked in the Amazon River, underwater. That was a thing that I invented. The piranha were about 30 feet away. I had a rope tied around me in case of attack, although people tell me now it would have been too late. I did

that for three hours and 40 minutes. It was scary, but fun."

At one time or another Furman has held the Guinness records for:

- Backwards unicycling: 53 miles
- Basketball dribbling in 24 hours: 83 miles
- Brick carrying (nine-pound brick in a one-handed pincer grip, palm down, walking): 64 miles
- Hopscotch (most games in 24 hours): 307
- Joggling 50 miles (juggling and running at the same time): 8 hours, 52 minutes
- Joggling marathon: 3 hours, 22 minutes
- Milk bottle balancing (glass bottle full of milk on the head): 70 miles
- Pogo-sticking: 15 miles
- Somersaults: 12¼ miles
- Squats, or deep knee-bends, in an hour: 4,495
- Step-ups in an hour (onto and off of a 15-inch exercise bench): 2,229

The Intuitive Workout

To keep in shape for these stunts, Furman exercises almost daily, but has no formal training schedule. "I'm very intuitive," he says. "My workouts revolve around whatever I'm training for. If I'm training for hopscotch, when I start getting into practices that last seven, eight or nine hours, then they take me quite a long time to recover. So I have

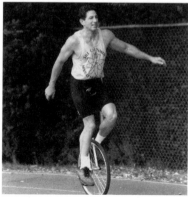

to work around that. I might work out with weights twice a week, run twice a week and jump rope. I also like rowing on a rowing machine."

Furman works toward a record with a slow-but-sure buildup, adding more repetitions each time he practices. "You look at that deep-knee-bend record and do 500," he says. " 'Wow, 500!' And the next time you do 600. It's progress you can see from day to day and week to week. The great thing is that the world is progressing, so you have to progress along with it. It would have been inconceivable for me to do 4,000 in an hour back in those days when the record was 1,800."

Furman has a flair for the exotic. The Guinness folks encourage sensational staging of events on the theory that it's hard to fake a record if there are thousands of witnesses and media coverage. Furman broke a knee-bend record in a hot-air balloon. He broke the walking-with-a-milk-bottle-on-your-head record in Indonesia and Switzerland. He broke the basketball dribbling record in Fiji. And he somer-saulted the entire length of Paul Revere's ride.

"The actual ride was Charlestown to Lexington," Furman says. "But I went the reverse because my friend told me the hills were more in my favor. It turns out they weren't. It was very hilly, and I got just as nauseous going down as going up."

No Limits

Furman was not always such a dynamo. He grew up with the name Keith and was the class nerd. In the 1970s he began studying Eastern philosophy and meditation under spiritual leader Sri Chinmoy, who gave him the name Ashrita, which means "Protected by God."

In 1978 Furman decided to join friends in a 24-hour bicycle race in Central Park. Using meditation techniques he had learned from Sri Chinmoy, he placed third out of thousands of participants, having ridden 405 miles.

"That was a major change, a major reve-

How He Does It	

The following is the training plan Ashrita Furman followed as he prepared to break the Guinness records for brick carrying and step-ups.

Monday

6:00–7:00 A.M.	meditation
8:00 A.M.	3-mile run on the streets

Tuesday

6:00–7:00 A.M.	meditation
8:00–8:30 A.M.	jumping rope
3:00–3:45 P.M.	weight lifting

Wednesday

6:00–7:00 A.M.	meditation
8:00–8:40 A.M.	jumping rope with high-speed intervals
3:00 P.M.	500 step-ups

Thursday

6:00–7:00 A.M.	meditation
8:00 A.M.	3-mile run
3:00–3:45 P.M.	weight lifting

Friday

6:00–7:00 A.M.	meditation
8:00–8:30 A.M.	jumping rope

Saturday

6:00–7:00 A.M.	meditation
10:00 A.M.–2 P.M.	brick carrying

Sunday

6:00–7:00 A.M.	meditation
8:00–10:00 A.M.	brick carrying around a track

lation for me—that anything is possible," he says. "If you can connect with your inner self you can do anything. There are no limits."

You Can Do It!

You don't need to be a professional athlete to be powerfully fit. These guys are the living proof. They face the same demands on their time as you, juggling jobs, families and other important factors. But they share a common commitment to peak conditioning. So can you.

Cycling through the Seasons

Dan Falk, Springfield, Pennsylvania

Date of birth: May 17, 1955

Height and weight: 5-foot-9, 175 pounds in the winter, 160 pounds in the summer

Profession: Computer consultant

I'm a cycling fanatic. That seems to be the overwhelming thing with me right now. But because I live in a cold-weather climate, I don't always get as much aerobic activity as I'd like in the winter. So I try to do more weight training and strengthening in the winter when I can't be outside running or riding a bike.

All year round, I do a split routine with weights, which means I don't try to exercise every body part on every trip to the gym. I'll typically work out in the winter four days a week with weights, and in the summer I may only get in two or three days a week. So in a split routine, I'll exercise biceps and back on one day; I'll do shoulders, chest and triceps on another day, and I'll concentrate on legs on a third day.

Because I rotate, I can go to the gym on consecutive days if I want and not worry about having to rest a certain muscle group. Because my schedule's hectic, I can't necessarily say, 'Oh gee, I can definitely go Monday, Wednesday and Friday.' But this way I *can* say,

'I better go Monday and Tuesday, because I don't know whether I can do it Thursday.'

I like the idea of working my legs in the winter rather than letting them just turn into total mush. I feel that I come out in the spring with some kind of base of strength that I might not have if I didn't train. I think weight training helps some in the swimming pool. And I'm a heck of a lot faster on the bike than I used to be, but I don't have 100 percent scientific proof that weights really translate into speed. Being stronger can't hurt, though—it has to help, and help you stay injury free.

So I have two phases of fitness: summer and winter. Year-round I lift weights. I swim, run, cycle, play tennis and hike. In the summer I'm active every day. In the winter I may miss two days a week. I'm less fit in the winter. I don't cycle much. I run some, but not enough. But I'm in the weight room, the swimming pool and on the indoor tennis courts more frequently. I weigh about 15 pounds more in the winter. My muscle mass is probably more in the winter as well, so it's not all fat.

There's a big split between my winter and summer diet, too. In the wintertime I tend to eat more heavily, probably more chicken and some red meat, as well as quite a few vegetables. In the summer I worry less in some ways, but I do worry about my fat intake. I think that's sort of the key thing to keeping weight off. If your diet isn't good, no amount of exercise is going to overcome that. I try to have fairly high fruit and vegetable intake. I try to avoid any kind of high-fat foods and lean more toward carbohydrates.

On the Road to Fitness

I've had my own computer business, Niagara Computer Services, for 12 years. I do programming and circuit design on a freelance basis. I also act as kind of a headhunter for temporaries. If I have more work than I can do, I'll try to place other consultants. This buys me a very large amount of personal flexibility. Sometimes in the summer I might go out at 3:00 P.M. and ride my bike for three hours or more, and if I have things I have to do, I can do them in the evening or early in the morning.

I pile on about 5,000 miles a year on a road bicycle. In late June every year I go to Colorado to cycle, and I participate in a thing called Ride the Rockies, which is sponsored by the Denver Post. That's usually about 420 miles over about a five- or six-day period at high elevations. And so I have to train substantially to be able to do that ride. I come out in late March, and I'll do 100 miles a week for maybe three weeks, and I start building up my mileage until I'm at a minimum of 150 miles a week. There's not much you can do to prepare for the elevation, but I find that the more fit you are, the less trouble you'll have.

I think you should try to do whatever you can to stay fit, even if that just means taking a walk for half an hour every day. That's true for me. I've come back from injuries where I could hardly do anything. I was hit by a car while I was riding my bike in Philadelphia in 1988. A taxicab blew a stop sign. I slammed on the brakes and crashed into the side of the cab. I had several broken ribs, and I had some internal bleeding. I had put my head through the window of the taxi cab but avoided serious head injury, probably because of my helmet.

How He Does It

This training schedule is typical of early June, preparing for the 420-mile Ride the Rockies in Colorado. Dan Falk rides 30 to 40 miles every weekday. All lifts are done pyramid-fashion: four sets, starting with lower weight and ten repetitions and ending with high weight and one to four repetitions, depending on the exercise. The schedule below is his sunny weather schedule. On rainy days, he substitutes biking with weight lifting and a 20-minute swim.

Monday

Weight lifting during lunch	(Shoulder, chest, triceps) Flat bench presses, incline bench presses, military presses, upright rows, dumbbell exercises for shoulders, narrow-grip bench presses, pull-downs, lying overhead triceps extensions

Wednesday

Weight lifting during lunch	(Back, biceps) Lat pull-downs and seated rows (both on machines), barbell curls with a straight bar, preacher curls with a curl bar

Saturday/Sunday

Bicycling	50–100 miles

I'm fine now, but I had to come back from being very out of shape. I would start out by just going for a walk. It's an incremental process: You can't go from being extremely out of shape to being in terrific shape overnight, and you have to start somewhere. Maybe that somewhere is just doing mild exercise and trying to cut down on fat intake.

Getting a Lift from Dancing

Dan Downing, Bethlehem, Pennsylvania

Date of birth: Dec. 10, 1959

Height and weight: 6 feet, 206 pounds

Profession: Banking officer

It sure didn't seem like it at the time, but when I broke my wrist in high school playing football with some friends, it turned out to be a lucky break. Otherwise, I might not have discovered the sport I love more than anything else I've ever done—power lifting and bodybuilding.

I had played football at the junior-high level, but just as I was starting high school, I had an unfortunate accident—suffering a severe break of my left wrist while playing a sandlot game. I was out for the year, and when you get behind a year or so while in rehabilitation, everyone else just keeps moving forward. So it's difficult to catch up. I started lifting weights to rebuild and strengthen my wrist, and really took a love to power lifting.

It got to the point where I wanted to compete with it. I joined the power-lifting team in the 165 pound class and usually placed in the top third in meets.

After high school I went right to work at Meridian Bank, which was then First National Bank of Allentown. It became more difficult to spend as much time in the gym, but I didn't stop lifting. Through the years I joined various area gyms and tried to stop in on Saturdays and some days after work.

Now, I work out at home. And my goals are different. I lift mainly to maintain physique and fitness. It isn't so much trying to do the biggest and heaviest lift. That's not that important anymore. Plus, it's very difficult to go really

heavy all the time. It's hard on your body, especially the power lifts.

I've been working out faithfully three to four times a week, from 45 minutes to 1½ hours. Most of the workouts I do are in the evening, after I get home from work. My weights are in the garage, and some nights, it's hard to go out there and lift. But I'm always glad when I do. If I come home from work and sit down on the sofa to watch TV, I find that if I haven't worked out, I wind up dozing off come 10:00 or 10:30. But if I work out, I usually will feel strong and refreshed.

I Could Have Danced All Night

My wife, Robin, and I have been married for almost nine years. When we first got married, we realized we had different interests. So we decided that we ought to try to come up with something that we could enjoy together, a mutual interest. I never dreamed it would be ballroom dancing. I didn't really dance much at all. But she talked me into it, and I'm glad she did. At first I felt self-conscious. But now, it's really enjoyable. I love it.

Plus, it's a great aerobic workout. If you jitterbug, which is something we really enjoy, and you're out there for a song that's several minutes long—whipping around and doing all kinds of intricate moves—when you're done with that dance, you're actually out of breath.

Looking and Feeling Good

Some people might consider bodybuilding vain, but it really isn't. I don't go around saying, "I lift weights. I'm a bodybuilder." But I'm proud of what I've done and of my physique. I feel better about myself.

I can't imagine ever quitting. In my senior years I would like to still be very physically fit. As we get older, certain areas of our bodies start to sag, or are not quite as tight

How He Does It

Monday

Barbell bench presses	3–4 sets, 6–8 reps
Alternating presses with dumbbells	3–4 sets, 6–8 reps
Dips	2 sets, 8–10 reps
Dumbbell flies	2–3 sets, 8–10 reps
Overhead extensions with curlbar	2 sets, 8–10 reps
Reverse grip triceps pull-downs on machine	2 sets, 10–12 reps
Kickbacks with dumbbells	2 sets, 10–12 reps

Tuesday

Regular chin-ups	3 sets, 6–8 reps
Lat pull-downs on machine (front)	3–4 sets, 8–12 reps
Lat pull-downs on machine (behind neck)	2 sets, 8–12 reps
Dumbbell rows	3 sets, 8–10 reps
Deadlifts with barbell	3 sets, 6–8 reps
Barbell curls (using curl bar)	3 sets, 8–10 reps
Dumbbell curls	2–3 sets, 8–10 reps

Thursday

Front lats with dumbbells	3 sets, 10–12 reps
Side lats with dumbbells	3 sets, 10–12 reps
Seated bent-over front raises	3 sets, 10–12 reps
Overhead extensions with barbell	2 sets, 6–8 reps
Bench presses with narrow grip (using curl bar)	2 sets, 6–8 reps
Triceps pull-downs on machine	2 sets, 6–8 reps
Standing high-pulley triceps extension	2 sets, 6–8 reps
Kickbacks with dumbbells	2 sets, 6–8 reps

Saturday

Squats	4 sets, 6–10 reps
Stiff-legged deadlifts with barbells	3 sets, 6–10 reps
Leg extensions	3 sets, 8–10 reps
Leg curls	3 sets, 8–10 reps

as they used to be. So it would be nice being an elderly man with a good physique. I think it would be appealing not only to me, but to my wife, Robin. I really believe that my reasons for lifting when I'm older will be the same reasons I do it now—fitness and physique.

Rock Hard at the Hard Rock Cafe

Scott Musgrave, Honolulu, Hawaii

Date of birth: July 3, 1962

Height and weight: 5-foot-11, 155 pounds

Profession: Head valet

As a college student, I loved spending my summers in Hawaii. I did all kinds of odd jobs to stay there—even parking cars at the Hard Rock Cafe. But when I was there those first summers, the one thing that really impressed me was how fitness-oriented everyone was. On any given weekend there was always some foot race or triathlon or swim race.

When I finished school, I settled down on the mainland to a corporate job—but that didn't interest me as much as the thought of living in Hawaii full-time. So, one day in 1990, I called up the boss at my old summer job at the Hard Rock and asked if I could work there for oh, about three months. I've been living on the island ever since, and I've really gotten into that fitness lifestyle everyone around here seems to enjoy. Now I'm head valet at the Hard Rock, and when I'm not doing that, I'm spending my time trying to keep my body rock hard. Since I moved here, I've competed in dozens of local triathlons and gradually worked my way up to the biggest of them all—the Ironman.

I first competed at Ironman level in 1994, doing the New Zealand race in February and then the one everybody knows—the Hawaii Ironman Triathlon on Kona, which I did in October of the same year. I admit, I wasn't close to winning or anything—the winner came in at something like 8:15, and I finished with 11:49. But just qualifying for the Ironman is an accomplishment in itself. We're talking about a race that combines swimming (2.4 miles), cycling (112 miles) and a marathon (26.2 miles). If you told me a few years ago that I'd be competing at that level, I never would have believed you. I guess I have my friends—and a good workout schedule—to thank for that.

In the beginning I had no real interest in the Ironman, but I did like cycling. When I moved to Hawaii, I brought my mountain bike with me and began riding the trails and roads on the island. And I did a little running, but nothing competitive—I just enjoyed being out there. Then a bunch of my friends got me into triathlon competition. I started doing one short race, then another and another. Boy, they were pretty miserable to do. Little by little, though, I started to improve—my form was getting better and my stamina wasn't so bad, either. And starting a regular workout routine was a big part of that.

Training in Paradise

Even in the off-season, I try to work out at least six days a week, usually seven. On at least four of those days, I get about an hour of weight training in. It's nothing special—I mix up free weights and circuit machines, and I work the basic muscle groups. I'm not trying to bulk up—it's just for a basic level of fitness. The main focus of my weekly routine is on the sports I'll need in competition—running, cycling and swimming.

Swimming's still my problem area—I need a lot of improvement, so I spend a lot of time during the week swimming with my masters' group. Monday, Wednesday and Friday, I swim at least 2000 meters under the watchful eye of my coach, Rowdy Gaines—he's the 1984 Olympic gold medalist in the 100-meter freestyle.

The rest of the week I run and cycle, covering a variety of terrains and distances. Off-season, a long run for me would be about 8 miles, but when I'm training, I work that up to 18. Cycling's the same story. Usually, I'll do at least 100 miles during the week, but during training, I'll do a 120-mile ride in a single day. And I'll mix up a lot of my rides with running immediately afterward. I'll round out the week with a long ride on Saturday, then a long run on Sunday.

All that work has really paid off. I went from not being much of a competitor to placing first in my age group in a number of smaller races and triathlons. And, of course, I've competed well enough in preliminaries to qualify for a spot in the Ironman.

Making Friends on the Road

But you know, as great as it is to earn a spot in the Ironman competition, the competition is not what it's all about for me. I don't have this cutthroat desire to win—I'm in there for the fun of it, too. When my friends got me into this—and I was having a tough time at first—having them around to encourage me really helped. It's that kind of social experience that draws me into the race. The shorter, local races are especially fun. The people are friendly, there's good food afterward and you get to make new friends. If you want to, you can even hook up with someone who's a little bit better than you, and that pushes you to be better. Not only do you have to keep up with them, but you can also learn some of their tricks. It's a great lifestyle.

And it's one I hope to pursue for a while. Because, when you think about it, it's really pretty ideal. I train early in the morning—I get to run and ride through some gorgeous landscape. Then I'll work an 11 to 5 shift or a 5 to midnight shift at the Hard Rock Cafe. It's a great gig, and it doesn't bite into my training schedule at all. It's a pretty carefree life. I'm single and selfish with my time right now, and that's pretty much how it is. I know I'm not going to do this forever, so I want to see how

How He Does It	
Monday	
Swimming	3000 meters
Tuesday	
Cycling	40–60 miles
(Rest)	
Distance running	4 miles early in season, gradually working up to 12 miles
Circuit and free weights	1 hour
Wednesday	
Swimming	3000 meters
Speed running	1 mile
Circuit and free weights	1 hour
Thursday	
Cycling	30–40 miles
Circuit and free weights	1 hour
Friday	
Swimming	3000 meters
Running (hilly terrain)	90 minutes
Circuit and free weights	1 hour
Saturday	
Cycling	100–120 miles
Sunday	
Distance running	16–18 miles

far I can go—how good I can get—while I can.

For the future I hope to keep getting stronger in the longer endurance events. I do pretty well in the short triathlons, but I need to make a breakthrough in my performance on the longer races like the Ironman. It's harder to sustain a powerful attitude for a longer race—in New Zealand, for example, my concentration wasn't all on the race. I have to be patient and work on that focus.

Working In the Workouts

Dan Sheehan, Lansdowne, Pennsylvania

Date of birth: Aug. 27, 1957

Height and weight: 5-foot-7, 172 pounds

Profession: Database technician/part-time musician

Some guys might think having five children, a wife and a job-and-a-half is workout enough. But for me, heading down to the basement to lift weights at home in the morning or squeezing in a workout on my lunch break isn't work—it's a labor of love. It's my time to recharge.

My wife, Becky, and I talk about this all the time. Every day, from the moment our feet hit the ground, we're running. Trying to get stuff done, trying to get the kids out the door. It's like the Keystone Cops here, especially in the mornings. Everything literally is down to the minute. We're going, going, going constantly.

And that's not including the time I spend with the band. I'm part of a duo called Two Guys. We sing and play guitar. Just two voices and two guitars. We play covers and swing tunes, and stuff like that. We've been together two years, and we're playing gigs all over the Philadelphia area, plus the coffeehouse circuit and the bookstore circuit. It's not easy. When you're done playing a few sets, you're exhausted. But I think I can do all this because I exercise so much. If you sit around all the time, you're tired. But when you push yourself and do your workouts, there's a certain spark that goes off. It sets a tone for your life so you don't have to come home from work and sit around on the sofa and watch television all night. You can get much more out of life.

Getting Creative

My time in the gym is time to reflect—especially during my morning workouts in the basement. Even though I'm working physically by lifting, I'm shut down and cut off from the world. For me it's a great way to start before I go off into the rhythm of the day. Everyone needs some type of reflection time—a time where you can turn things off a little bit.

It's funny, but even when I'm downstairs working out and I need to rest between sets, I can still get things done. It's like I have more energy. I can read something in between sets or catch up on things. I've even done things as wild as doing a set of lifting downstairs and then running upstairs to start a load of wash.

My approach to lifting is simple. It's definitely unscientific. I mean, my equipment at home is really minimal. All I have is a bench, 350 pounds of plates, an Olympic bar and a curling bar. So let's just say I've learned to be creative. For example, instead of dumbbell work—since I don't have dumbbells—I'll use plates instead. For front lateral raises for my shoulders, I'll hold two 11-pound plates and do 25 reps. It works the shoulders, plus it builds grip strength.

I can see and feel the changes. My arms and chest have gotten bigger, and I can look in the mirror and think, "Wow, this stuff really does work."

Walking To Fitness

The weakest link in my workout—besides being strapped for time—is my abs. I probably don't spend as much time on them as I should. But I do pay attention to aerobic conditioning and nutrition. I walk 2½ miles to the train station every morning wearing a heavy backpack. I fill my pack with my office stuff, my lunch and my gym bag, and I hoof it to the terminal. It's a conscious effort to get some aerobic conditioning, and I do it in all sorts of weather. Barring anything that would break my neck, like the few times in the winter when everything's a sheet of ice, I walk every day.

As for nutrition, again I'm not really scientific. I could stand to learn a lot more, but I do watch my fat intake. And I don't drink alcohol anymore. I cheat sometimes at the food. I'm a human being, so I'm not perfect. But I have switched to drinking skim milk and eating lots of cereal. I also eat lots of tuna, pasta and chicken. Becky's been a big factor in this, because now we'll buy low-fat lunch meats, and instead of ordering out for a pizza, we'll get the kids and make our own pizza using low-fat mozzarella cheese. It's not as caustic as going out to a pizza joint.

Working out has been a really positive thing in my life. When I first got married 15 years ago, I was pushing 200 pounds. I didn't exercise at all, and I ate all the wrong foods. I also drank a lot. I had been flirting with going to the gym periodically; then one day around 1989, I took up running. I'd do six or seven miles at a clip, and the longest I ever ran was 13 miles in the Philadelphia Half Marathon. When I was introduced to weight lifting by some regular lifters I knew, something clicked. Especially when I started seeing results.

Now, after a good workout, I feel great. The endorphins are pumping and I feel fine. Of course, two hours later I want to take a nap, but that's okay. It's worth the effort I put into it. I look at some of the guys I went to high school with, and I know I'm in much better shape than they are. That's part of the appeal of weight lifting: You can see what it does for you. It not only makes you feel better—and I do feel better—but it's something you can do for your body that's constructive.

How He Does It

Monday/Wednesday/Friday

6:00 A.M. workout at home:

Oblique twists (with a broomstick)	1–2 sets, 100 reps
Crunches	1–2 sets, 50–100 reps
Bench presses (warm-up)	1 set, 20 reps
(add weight)	4 sets, 4 reps
(decrease weight)	4 sets, 13 reps
Curls (warm-up)	3 sets, 12 reps
(add weight)	3 sets, 10 reps
Upright rows	3 sets, 10–12 reps

Lunchtime workout:

Dumbbell flies	4 sets, 6 reps
Dumbbell pull-overs	4 sets, 10–12 reps
Lat pull-downs	2 sets, 14 reps
(add weight)	2 sets, 10 reps
Triceps pull-downs	2 sets, 10 reps

Tuesday/Thursday

6:00 A.M. workout at home:

Curls	1 set, 7 reps
(partials)	1 set, 7 reps
(partials)	1 set, 7 reps
Triceps extensions	3 sets, 12 reps

Lunchtime workout:

Squats (warm-up)	1 set, 14 reps
(add weight)	3 sets, 10 reps
(add weight)	3 sets, 8 reps
Leg extensions	2 sets, 13 reps
Leg curls	2 sets, 12 reps

Sunday

More than an hour of mixed Monday/Tuesday schedule

Index

Note: **Boldface** references indicate primary discussion of topic.